中英日對照
實用針灸手册

PRACTICAL HANDBOOK ON ACUPUNCTURE AND MOXIBUSTION

実用針灸ハンドブック

安西川　陳方良　張玉娟　編著

吉林科學技術出版社

First Edition 1989

Practical Handbook on Acupuncture and Moxibustion

by

An Xichuan Chen Fangliang Zhang Yujuan
Published by
Jilin Science and Technology Press
102 Stalin Street, Changchun, China
Printed by
Changchun Xinhua Printing House
23 Jilin Road, Changchun, China
Distributed by
China International Book Trading Corporation
(GUOJI SHUDIAN)
P. O. Box. 399, Beijing, China
ISBN 7-5384-0351-5/R·58
Printed in the People's Republic of China

如何运用外国的语言正确地翻译表达我国针灸学的真正涵义，这是当今我们适应世界出现"针灸热"的一个十分重大的课题。我衷心希望吉林省中医研究院安西川教授等所编写的这部中英日对照《实用针灸手册》能够实现这个目的。

中国卫生部副部长
国家中医药管理局局长　胡熙明

一九八八年七月十日

序

针灸学是祖国医学的重要组成部分，是我国广大人民数千年来与疾病作斗争的经验总结，是医学中灿烂的瑰宝，已为世界各国人民所瞩目。

针灸疗法以其奏效神速，适应症广，用具简单，操作方便为特色，故深为广大群众所喜爱。

中华人民共和国成立以来，我国的针灸无论在经络的理论研究方面，或在临床的实践方面，都有很大进展。近年来随着对外政策的开放，各国朋友纷纷前来我国学习针灸技术或接受针灸治疗。国内医务工作者越来越多地使用或配合针灸疗法，提高了医疗效果。援外医疗队用针灸疗法，收到显著的疗效，给国外人士以深刻的印象。据不完全统计，现在已经有120多个国家或地区有了自己的针灸医生。在世界范围内，一个学习、应用和研究针灸的热潮方兴未艾。1987年11月25日在中国北京，正式成立了世界针灸学会联合会。我们高兴地看到，源于我国、具有悠久历史的针灸医学已经成为世界医学的一个重要组成部分，正在为人类健康事业发挥着日益重要的作用。为适应国内外针灸爱好者的迫切需要，编著一本简明易学的手册，实为当前之急务。

吉林省中医中药研究院安西川教授、陈方良教授以及白求恩医科大学张玉娟讲师，以其多年对针灸、中医、外语等讲学的经验，特别是结合对国际友人举办的针灸学习班讲学的经验，合力编写中英日对照《实用针灸手册》一书，该书以简练的文字，用中英日三种语言，采取分段互为对照的方式，重点地介绍了针灸基础理论，临床常用的96个腧穴的定位，主治和操作，50种临床常见病的处方和配穴，并附有验案，还有和针灸临床有关的

英日文常用语和常用词汇。可谓用心周到,照顾全面,易学易用。既可作为国际友人学习针灸的教材,又可作为我出国医务人员的必携资料,还可作为医科学生学习专业外语的参考。这对我国针灸医学对外交流,将起到积极的促进作用。

张继有
1989年元月

Foreword

Acupuncture and moxibustion are important components of Chinese traditional medicine, and a summary of experience by ordinary Chinese people to the struggle against disease over thousands of years. As valuable contributions to medicine, acupuncture and moxibustion are the focus of people's attention from all parts of the world.

These techniques are characterized by their amazingly rapid attainment of the desired results, their wide indications, and the simple equipment and easy manipulation required. They have therefore been widely accepted by the general population.

Acupuncture and moxibustion in China have made considerable progress, both in the theoretical study of channels and collaterals and in clinical practice since the founding of the People's Republic of China. In recent years, with foreign policy becoming more open, numerous visitors from various countries have come to China to study acupuncture and moxibustion techniques and to accept treatment with acupuncture and moxibustion. In China, medical workers have increasingly made use of acupuncture and moxibustion therapy and have incorporated these techniques alongside western medicine to raise the effectiveness of medical treatment. Remarkable therapeutic results, which have left a deep impression on foreigners, have been achieved by Chinese medical teams working to aid foreign countries. According to incomplete statistics, more than 120 countries and regions across the world have their own acupuncture and moxibustion doctors. A great upsurge in the application and study of acupuncture and moxibustion is now in the ascendant all over the world. The World Federation of Acupuncture and Moxibustion Societies (WFAS) was formally set up on November 25, 1987, in Beijing, China. We are glad to see that acupuncture and moxibustion, with an ancient history originating in China, have become an essential component of world medicine, providing a great service for human health and playing an increasingly important role in the world. In order to satisfy the urgent needs of those, at home and abroad, who are in favor of acupuncture and moxibustion, a simple, clear and easy-to-study handbook was necessary to be edited by us.

Prof. An Xichuan and Chen Fangliang of Jilin Provincial Academy of Traditional Chinese Medicine and Material Medica and Lecturer Zhang Yujuan of Norman Bethune University of Medical Sciences have pooled efforts to compile a Chinese-English-Japanese trilingual «Practical Handbook on Acupuncture and Moxibustion». This is based on our experience of teaching acupuncture and moxibustion, traditional Chinese medicine and foreign languages in recent years, combined with practical teaching experience in acupuncture and moxibustion courses for foreign colleagues. Concisely written, in Chinese, English, and Japanese, the book briefly introduces the key points of t... of acupuncture and moxibustion. The 96 ...ory used acupuncture points and the prescriptions and ...y nation of points for 50 common diseases are introdu... There is an appendix with examples of typical cases. The book also introduces sentences and an English and Japanese glossary of special terms commonly used in the clinical practice of acupuncture and moxibustion. Care is taken to edit this book for easily studying and varied application. This book may be used as a textbook for acupuncture and moxibustion study by foreign practitioners, as an indispensable aid for medical workers who go abroad, and as a reference book for practical foreign language study by medical students. The book will play an active role in facilitating external exchanges.

Zhang Jiyou
January, 1989.

序

　針灸学は中国医学の重要な構成部分をなし、中国の広はんな人民が幾千年来、疾病と闘い人民に貢献してきた医学の中でも、他に類をみない傑出した独特な医術であり、今や国際的にも注目の的となっているものである。
　針灸療法は、即効性があり、適応症が広く、大掛りな設備を必要とせず、操作も簡単であるなど数数の特色があり、多くの人人に深く浸透している。
　中華人民共和国が成立して以来、中国の針灸は、飛躍的な発展をとげてきた。特にここ数年来、中国の対外開放政策により、各国から数多くの人人が針灸医術の学習、あるいは針灸治療を受けるために中国を訪れている。中国の医療関係者が、ますます針灸を総合療法として用いることが多くなり、治療効果を、より一層高めるところとなった。中国の対外援助医療隊も針灸療法によって、顕著な効果をあげ、外国の人人に強い感銘を与えた。不完全な統計ではあるが、世界120個国余の国家、あるいは地域に針灸医がおり、針灸の学習、応用、研究が世界的なひろまりをみせ、高い評価をうけてきている。1987年11月25日中国の北京において、世界針灸学会連合会が正式に成立した。この事実は非常に意義のあることであり、又喜ばしいことである。すなわち、このことは、中国に起源をもち、数千年の歴史を有する針灸医学が今日世界に向かって大きく発展し、世界の医学にとって不可欠な構成要素となり、人類の疾病治療と保健に、ますます重要な位置をしめ、針灸が大きな力を発揮していることを示している。以上の情勢にこたえるため、針灸を

学習する者にとって、きわめて便利で、内容が平易にして、要を得た、針灸ハンドブックを作成することが我我の急務であると考える。

　吉林省中医中薬研究院の安西川教授、陳方良教授、白求恩医科大学の張玉娟講師らが、多年の針灸、漢方医学と外国語の講義経験、特に外国人の針灸研修のために講義をした経験を基に、中英日対照「実用針灸ハンドブック」として本書を編著した。簡潔な文章で、中英日の三個国語を対照して、理解しやすく、且つ要点をつかむことを目的に、針灸の基本理論、操作方法、常用穴96個、臨床でよく見かける疾病50種などを紹介し、さらに症例解説を附している。また針灸臨床によく用いる英語、日本語と単語集をのせ、学習にも、実用にも、最も適切で、外国人のよい針灸学習教材であると同時に、中国の対外援助医療隊員の必携資料にもなることに主眼をおき、あわせて医学生が専門外国語を学習するための参考書ともなるものであることに心掛けた。必ずや中国針灸医学の国際的交流を、さらに一層推進し、針灸医学の発展に貢献できるものと確信している。

張継有
1989年1月

前　言

　　本书以中、英、日三种文字对照，分为上、中、下三篇。上篇着重介绍针灸操作方法，经络和96个常用腧穴；中篇则以针灸治疗的处方与配穴原则为指导，介绍了50种常见病的临床治疗，并附有验案15例；下篇介绍与针灸临床有关的英、日文常用语100句及常用词汇。

　　本书承蒙世界针灸学会联合会主席、中国卫生部副部长、中国中医药管理局局长胡熙明同志题词。承蒙吉林省中医中药研究院名誉院长张继有教授作序和审阅。本书英文部分由白求恩医科大学吕文赏教授全面审阅，并请英国生物学医学科学作家伍德豪斯先生作了部分审阅；日文部分由日本国长野县中国鍼创建会中医研究所院长、吉林省中医中药研究院客座副研究员草间秀夫先生及白求恩医科大学邹元植教授全面审阅，在此深致谢意。

　　本书的编写出版，得到了吉林省卫生厅副厅长刘庆欣教授，以及吉林省中医管理局、吉林省卫生厅科教处同志的鼓励和支持，在此一并致谢。

　　本书由安西川教授组织编写，英语部分由张玉娟讲师执笔，日语部分由陈方良教授执笔。由于编者的水平所限，加之时间仓促，不足之处，敬请惠予指正。

编　者
1989年2月

Preface

This book is written in three languages, Chinese, English and Japanese for introducing Chinese acupuncture and moxibustion to the world. It Consists of three parts. Part A introduces the techniques of acupuncture and moxibustion, the channels and collaterals, and 96 commonly used acupuncture points. Part B deals with the clinical treatment of 50 common diseases with an appendix of 15 examples of typical cases for acupuncture and moxibustion therapy, which is guided by the principles governing the prescription and combination of points of acupuncture and moxibustion therapy. Part C introduces 100 sentences and glossary of special terms commonly used in English and Japanese in the clinical practice of acupuncture and moxibustion.

The wonderful inscription on the book for congratulation isw ritten by Mr. Hu Ximing, Chairman of the World Federation of Acupuncture and Moxibustion Societies, Chinese Vice-Minister of Public Health, Head of the State Traditional Medical Science Administration of the PRC. The introduction of this book is given by Prof. Zhang Jiyou, Honorary Dean of Jilin Provincial Academy of Traditional Chinese Medicine and Material Medica and he also reads the manuscript through. We express our thanks to Prof. Lü Wenshang of Norman Bethune University of Medical Sciences for her helpful suggestions of the Eng-

...ipt and Mr. R. J. Woodhouse MSc. an English medical science writer, for the reading of one of the English manuscript. We are greatly indebted Mr. Hideo Kusama, Dean of Traditional Chinese Medical Institute of Sōken Society in Nagano Prefecture, Japan, and guest associate research fellow of Jilin Provincial Academy of Traditional Chinese Medicine and Material Medica, and Prof. Zou Yuanzhi of Norman Bethune University of Medicel Sciences for reading the Japanese manuscript.

Acknowledgement must be made to Prof. Liu Qingxin, a Deputy Director of Jilin Provincial Health Bureau, Jilin Provincial Traditional Medical Science Administration and the Scientific Education Office of Jilin Provincial Health Bureau for their great encouragement and support in the compilation and publication.

This book is edited by Prof. An Xichuan, the English part by Ms. Zhang Yujuan, the Japanese part by Prof. Chen Fangliang. We wish to thank readers for their coming criticism and suggestions. These will always be welcome.

authors.
February, 1989.

はじめに

　このハンドブックは、中国語、英語、日本語の三ケ国語を対照させ、上、中、下の三篇に分けられている。上篇では、針灸の操作方法、経絡と臨床によく使用する腧穴の穴位96個を紹介し、中篇では、針灸治療の処方と配穴の原則にもとづき、50種のよく見かける疾病を紹介して、15例の症例解説を附している、下篇では、針灸治療の臨床によく使用する言葉100句と英語、日本語の単語を紹介している。

　編さんするにあたって、題字して下さった世界針灸学会連合会主席、中国衞生部副部長、国家中医薬管理局局長胡熙明先生。全文を詳しく検討、校閲し、序文を書いて下さった吉林省中医中薬研究院名誉院長張継有教授。英語の部分を詳しく校閲して下さった白求恩医科大学の呂文賞教授、イギリスの生物と医学科学作家ウード・ホース先生、日本語の部分を全面に校閲して下さった日本国長野県中国鍼創建会中医研究所院長、吉林省中医中薬研究院客座副研究員草間秀夫先生と白求恩医科大学の鄒元植教授に深甚なる感謝の意を表する次第である。

　なお、このハンドブックの出版を支持し、激励して下さった吉林省衞生庁副庁長劉慶欣教授、ならびに吉林省中医管理局、吉林省衞生庁科研教育処の諸先生方に厚く御礼申し上げる。

　このハンドブックの編さんは、安西川教授が監修、執筆し、張玉娟講師は英語部分、陳方良教授は日本語部分を分担執筆した。編さんに必ずしも充分な時間をとることができなかったことは残念であるが、本書の目的は、針灸の学習と臨床に最も

適切で、理解しやすいところにある。多多ゆきとどかないところもあるかと思うが、所期の目的を達成てきたら、この上ない喜びである。

編 者
1989年2月

目 录

上篇 针灸的基本知识

第一章 什么是针灸疗法 ……………………（ 3 ）
第二章 针灸疗法的优点 ……………………（ 4 ）
第三章 针灸法 ………………………………（ 8 ）
  第一节 针法 ………………………………（ 8 ）
  第二节 灸法 ………………………………（ 25 ）
  〔附〕拔罐疗法 …………………………（ 28 ）
第四章 经络与腧穴 …………………………（ 30 ）
  第一节 分类及分布 ………………………（ 30 ）
  第二节 腧穴的定位法 ……………………（ 33 ）
  第三节 十四经脉与腧穴 …………………（ 40 ）
    1. 手太阴肺经 …………………………（ 40 ）
      列缺 太渊 鱼际 少商
    2. 手阳明大肠经 ………………………（ 45 ）
      商阳 合谷 曲池 肩髃 迎香
    3. 足阳明胃经 …………………………（ 51 ）
      地仓 颊车 下关 头维 梁门 天枢 伏兔
      梁丘 犊鼻 足三里 丰隆 解溪 内庭 厉兑
    4. 足太阴脾经 …………………………（ 65 ）
      隐白 三阴交 阴陵泉 血海
    5. 手少阴心经 …………………………（ 70 ）
      通里 神门 少冲
    6. 手太阳小肠经 ………………………（ 74 ）
      少泽 后溪 肩贞 天宗 听宫
    7. 足太阳膀胱经 ………………………（ 80 ）
      睛明 攒竹 肺俞 心俞 膈俞 肝俞

　　　　脾俞　肾俞　秩边　委中　承山　昆仑　至阴

　8. 足少阴肾经 …………………………………………（93）
　　　　涌泉　太溪　照海　复溜

　9. 手厥阴心包经 ………………………………………（98）
　　　　间使　内关　劳宫　中冲

　10. 手少阳三焦经 ………………………………………（103）
　　　　中渚　外关　支沟　翳风　耳门

　11. 足少阳胆经 …………………………………………（108）
　　　　瞳子髎　听会　阳白　风池　带脉　环跳　风市
　　　　阳陵泉　悬钟　足窍阴

　12. 足厥阴肝经 …………………………………………（119）
　　　　行间　太冲　期门

　13. 督脉 …………………………………………………（123）
　　　　长强　命门　大椎　风府　百会　上星　人中

　14. 任脉 …………………………………………………（130）
　　　　中极　关元　气海　中脘　膻中　天突　廉泉　承浆

　15. 经外奇穴 ……………………………………………（138）
　　　　四神聪　印堂　太阳　金津　玉液　十宣　华佗夹脊

中篇　针灸的临床治疗

　第五章　处方配穴的基本原则 ……………………………（149）
　第六章　常见病证的针灸治疗 ……………………………（154）
　　感冒 …………………………………………………………（154）
　　咳嗽 …………………………………………………………（156）
　　喘证 …………………………………………………………（159）
　　中暑 …………………………………………………………（162）
　　呃逆 …………………………………………………………（163）
　　呕吐 …………………………………………………………（165）
　　泄泻 …………………………………………………………（167）
　　便秘 …………………………………………………………（170）
　　痢疾 …………………………………………………………（172）
　　胃脘痛 ………………………………………………………（175）
　　黄疸 …………………………………………………………（177）

水肿	(179)
淋证	(181)
癃闭	(183)
遗尿	(185)
阳痿	(186)
遗精	(188)
中风	(189)
口眼歪斜	(193)
头痛	(195)
眩晕	(197)
心悸、怔忡	(200)
癫狂	(202)
不寐	(205)
胁痛	(207)
腹痛	(209)
腰痛	(211)
痹证	(214)
痿证	(216)
扭挫伤	(219)
脏躁	(221)
崩漏	(223)
痛经	(225)
闭经	(227)
带下	(229)
妊娠恶阻	(230)
胎位不正	(232)
乳汁少	(234)
小儿惊风	(235)
小儿腹泻	(237)
耳鸣耳聋	(239)
目赤肿痛	(241)
齿痛	(242)

咽喉肿痛	（244）
鼻衄	（245）
风疹	（247）
缠腰火丹	（248）
疔疮	（250）
气瘿	（252）
消渴	（254）
〔附〕典型病例介绍	（256）

第七章 耳针疗法 （277）

第一节 耳与经络、脏腑的关系 （278）
第二节 耳针的穴位 （281）
第三节 耳针的临床应用 （282）

下篇 针灸诊疗常用语及词汇

第一节 常用语 （295）
第二节 词汇 （313）
　〔附〕中文简化字繁体字对照 （371）

Contents

PART A An Elementary Description of Acupuncture and Moxibustion

  Chapter Ⅰ What Acupuncture and Moxibustion Therapy Is ······ (3)

  Chapter Ⅱ The Advantages of Acupuncture and Moxibustion Therapy ············· (5)

  Chapter Ⅲ The Techniques of Acupuncture and Moxibustion ······················· (10)

    Ⅰ. Manipulation of the Needle ················ (10)

    Ⅱ. Moxibustion ··· (26)

      〔Appendix〕 Cupping ···························· (28)

  Chapter Ⅳ Channels, Collaterals and Points ··· (31)

    Ⅰ. Classification and Distribution ·············· (31)

    Ⅱ. Methods for Locating Points ················ (33)

    Ⅲ. The 14 Regular Channels and Their Points ··· (40)

      1. The Lung Channel of Hand-Taiyin ········ (40)
        Lieque Taiyuan Yuji Shaoshang

      2. The Large Intestine Channel of Hand-Yangming ································ (45)
        Shangyang Hegu Quchi Jianyu Yingxiang

      3. The Stomach Channel of Foot-Yangming ······································· (51)
        Dicang Jiache Xiaguan Touwei Liangmen
        Tianshu Futu Liangqiu Dubi Zusanli
        Fenglong Jiexi Neiting Lidui

...n Channel of Foot-Taiyin .... (65)
   ...ai Sanyinjiao Yinlingquan Xuehai
   ...e Heart Channel of Hand-Shaoyin .... (70)
   Tongli Shenmen Shaochong

6. The Small Intestine Channel of Hand-
   Taiyang .... (74)
   Shaoze Houxi Jianzhen Tianzong Tinggong

7. The Urinary Bladder Channel of
   Foot-Taiyang .... (80)
   Jingming Zanzhu Feishu Xinshu Geshu
   Ganshu Pishu Shenshu Zhibian Weizhong
   Chengshan Kunlun Zhiyin

8. The Kidney Channel of Foot-Shaoyin .... (93)
   Yongquan Taixi Zhaohai Fuliu

9. The Pericardium Channel of Hand-
   Jueyin .... (98)
   Jianshi Neiguan Laogong Zhongchong

10. The Sanjiao Channel of Hand-
    Shaoyang .... (103)
    Zhongzhu Waiguan Zhigou Yifeng
    Ermen

11. The Gall Bladder Channel of Foot-
    Shaoyang .... (108)
    Tongziliao Tinghui Yangbai Fengchi
    Daimai Huantiao Fengshi Yanglingquan
    Xuanzhong Foot-Qiaoyin

12. The Liver Channel of Foot-Jueyin .... (119)
    Xingjian Taichong Qimen

13. The Du Channel .... (123)
    Changqiang Mingmen Dazhui Fengfu
    Baihui Shangxing Renzhong

14. The Ren Channel .... (130)
    Zhongji Guanyuan Qibai Zhongwan

      Shanzhong Tiantu Lianquan Chengjiang
  15. Extraordinary Points .... (138)
      Sishencong Yintang Taiyang Jinjin Yuye
      Shixuan Huatuo Jiaji

PART B   Clinical Therapy of Acupuncture and Moxibustion

  Chapter V   The Basic Principles Governing Prescription and Combination of Points .... (149)

  Chapter VI   Treatment of Common Diseases with Acupuncture and Moxibustion ... (154)

      The Common Cold .... (155)
      Cough .... (157)
      Asthma .... (160)
      Sunstroke .... (162)
      Hiccup .... (164)
      Vomiting .... (166)
      Diarrhea .... (168)
      Constipation .... (171)
      Dysentery .... (173)
      Epigastric Pain .... (175)
      Jaundice .... (177)
      Edema .... (179)
      Stranguria .... (181)
      Retention of Urine .... (183)
      Nocturnal Enuresis .... (185)
      Impotence .... (187)
      Seminal Emission .... (188)
      Windstroke .... (190)
      Facial Paralysis .... (193)
      Headache .... (196)

Dizziness and Vertigo .... (198)
Palpitation, Anxiety .... (200)
Depressive and Manic Mental Disorders ...... (203)
Insomnia .... (206)
Hypochondriac Pain .... (208)
Abdominal Pain .... (210)
Low Back Pain .... (212)
Bi Syndrome .... (214)
Wei Syndrome .... (217)
Sprain .... (220)
Hysteria .... (222)
Uterine Hemorrhage .... (224)
Dysmenorrhea .... (226)
Amenorrhea .... (227)
Leukorrhea .... (229)
Morning Sickness .... (231)
Abnormal Position of Fetus .... (232)
Lactation Insufficiency .... (234)
Infantile Convulsion .... (236)
Infantile Diarrhea .... (238)
Deafness and Tinnitus .... (239)
Congestion, Swelling and Pain of the Eye ...... (241)
Toothache .... (243)
Sore Throat .... (244)
Epistaxis .... (246)
Urticaria .... (247)
Herpes Zoster .... (249)
Furuncle .... (250)
Goiter .... (252)
Emaciation-Thirst Diseases .... (254)
[Appendix] Examples of Typical Cases ...... (256)

Chapter Ⅶ　Ear Acupuncture Therapy ············ (277)
　Ⅰ. Relations between the Auricle and
　　　Channels, Collaterals and Zang-Fu
　　　Organs ·· (279)
　Ⅱ. Auricular Points ······························ (281)
　Ⅲ. Clinical Application of Ear
　　　Acupuncture ······································ (284)

PART C Sentences and Glossary Commonly Used in Acupuncture and Moxibustion during the Consultation Procedure

　Ⅰ. Common Sentences ·························· (295)
　Ⅱ. Glossary ·· (313)

目 次

上篇 針灸の基本知識
第一章 針灸療法とは ……………………………………（ 4 ）
第二章 針灸療法の利点 …………………………………（ 5 ）
第三章 針灸法 ……………………………………………（ 11 ）
第一節 毫針の刺し方 …………………………………（ 11 ）
第二節 灸法 ……………………………………………（ 26 ）
〔附〕抜罐療法 ………………………………………（ 29 ）

第四章 経絡と腧穴………………………………………（ 32 ）
第一節 分類及び分布 …………………………………（ 32 ）
第二節 腧穴の定位法 …………………………………（ 34 ）
第三節 十四経脈と腧穴 ………………………………（ 40 ）
1. 手の太陰肺経 …………………………………………（ 41 ）
   列缺 太淵 魚際 少商
2. 手の陽明大腸経 ………………………………………（ 46 ）
   商陽 合谷 曲池 肩髃 迎香
3. 足の陽明胃経 …………………………………………（ 53 ）
   地倉 頰車 下関 頭維 梁門 天枢 伏兎
   梁丘 犢鼻 足三里 豊隆 解谿 内庭 厲兌
4. 足の太陰脾経 …………………………………………（ 65 ）
   隠白 三陰交 陰陵泉 血海
5. 手の少陰心経 …………………………………………（ 71 ）
   通里 神門 少衝
6. 手の太陽小腸経 ………………………………………（ 75 ）
   少沢 後谿 肩貞 天宗 聴宮
7. 足の太陽膀胱経 ………………………………………（ 80 ）
   睛明 攅竹 肺俞 心俞 膈俞 肝俞 脾俞 腎俞

　　　　　秩辺　委中　承山　崑崙　至陰
　　8. 足の少陰腎経 ……………………………………（ 93 ）
　　　　　湧泉　太谿　照海　復溜
　　9. 手の厥陰心包経 …………………………………（ 98 ）
　　　　　間使　内関　労宮　中衝
　　10. 手の少陽三焦経 …………………………………（ 103 ）
　　　　　中渚　外関　支溝　翳風　耳門
　　11. 足の少陽胆経 ……………………………………（ 108 ）
　　　　　瞳子髎　聴会　陽白　風池　帯脈　環跳
　　　　　風市　陽陵泉　懸鐘　足竅陰
　　12. 足の厥陰肝経 ……………………………………（ 119 ）
　　　　　行間　太衝　期門
　　13. 督脈 ………………………………………………（ 123 ）
　　　　　長強　命門　大椎　風府　百会　上星　人中
　　14. 任脈 ………………………………………………（ 130 ）
　　　　　中極　関元　気海　中脘　膻中　天突　廉泉　承漿
　　15. 経外奇穴 …………………………………………（ 138 ）
　　　　　四神聡　印堂　太陽　金津　玉液　十宣　華陀夾脊

中篇　針灸の臨床治療

第五章　処方配穴の基本原則 ……………………（ 150 ）
第六章　よく見かける病症の針灸治療 …………（ 154 ）

　　感冒 …………………………………………（ 155 ）
　　咳嗽 …………………………………………（ 158 ）
　　喘息 …………………………………………（ 161 ）
　　日射病 ………………………………………（ 163 ）
　　吃逆 …………………………………………（ 165 ）
　　嘔吐 …………………………………………（ 167 ）
　　下痢 …………………………………………（ 169 ）
　　便秘 …………………………………………（ 172 ）
　　細菌性下痢 …………………………………（ 174 ）
　　胃脘痛 ………………………………………（ 176 ）
　　黄疸 …………………………………………（ 178 ）

項目	頁
水腫	(180)
淋症	(182)
癃閉	(184)
遺尿	(186)
陰萎	(187)
遺精	(189)
卒中	(192)
口眼歪邪	(194)
頭痛	(197)
眩暈	(199)
心悸、怔忡	(201)
癲狂	(204)
不眠	(207)
脇痛	(209)
腹痛	(211)
腰痛	(213)
痺症	(215)
萎症	(218)
捻挫傷	(220)
臟躁	(222)
崩漏	(224)
生理痛	(226)
月經閉止	(228)
帶下	(230)
妊娠惡阻	(231)
胎位不正	(233)
乳汁分泌不足	(235)
小兒驚風	(236)
小兒下痢	(238)
耳鳴、難聽	(240)
目赤腫痛	(242)
齒痛	(243)

咽喉腫痛 ……………………………………（245）
　　　鼻血 ………………………………………（246）
　　　風疹 ………………………………………（248）
　　　纏腰火丹 …………………………………（249）
　　　疔瘡 ………………………………………（251）
　　　気瘻 ………………………………………（253）
　　　消渇 ………………………………………（255）
　　　〔附〕症例解説 …………………………（256）
　第七章　耳針療法 …………………………（278）
　　第一節　耳と経絡・臟腑との関係 ………（280）
　　第二節　耳針の穴位 ………………………（282）
　　第三節　耳針の臨床応用 …………………（285）

下篇　針灸の診断治療に常用する言葉およひ単語

　　第一節　常用する言葉 ……………………（295）
　　第二節　単語 ………………………………（348）

上篇 针灸的基本知识

PART A An Elementary Description of Acupuncture and Moxibustion

上篇 針灸の基本知識

上篇 针灸的基本知识

PART A An Elementary Description of Acupuncture and Moxibustion

上篇 针灸①基本知篇

第一章 什么是针灸疗法

针法和灸法是两种不同的治疗方法。针法是采用各种不同型号的金属针,通过刺入穴位进行治病的方法;灸法是主要采用艾叶制成的艾绒,点燃后,通过熏灼腧穴或部位进行治病的方法。两者所用的器材和操作方法虽不相同,但都是通过刺激人体的经络和腧穴而起到疏通经络、调和气血的作用,从而达到防治疾病的目的。在临床上,针法和灸法常结合使用,故通称为针灸疗法。

Chapter I What Acupuncture and Moxibustion Therapy Is

Acupuncture and moxibustion are two distinct therapeutic methods. Acupuncture treats disease by puncturing certain points of the human body with different types of metal needles, while moxibustion is the application of heat produced by ignited moxa-wool made from dry moxa leaves over the points of the skin surface or certain locations in the human body. Although the equipments and materials used in the two methods are different, the therapeutic and preventive results in both cases are similarly achieved i.e. through promoting smooth circulation of the channels and adjusting qi (氣) and blood (血) by stimulating the points and channels, thus achieving the aim of prevention and treatment of diseases. Clinically, acupuncture and moxibustion methods are frequently used combinedly and are therefore known as acupuncture and moxibustion therapy.

第一章　針灸療法とは

　針と灸は二つの異なる治療方法である。針法とは金属で作った一定の規格の針具で、人体の穴位に刺し入れ、疾病を治療する方法である。灸法とは、一定の形状のもぐさを燃やして、腧穴あるいは人体のある部位に、温熱の刺激をあたえて、疾病を治療する方法である。この二つの方法に用いる器具と操作方法は違うが、いずれも人体の経絡と腧穴を刺激して、経絡を疏通させ、気血を調節する作用により、疾病の預防と治療する目的に達するものである。臨床において、針法と灸法をよく組み合わせて行うので、普通は針灸療法と称する。

第二章　针灸疗法的优点

　针灸疗法是中国几千年来一直深受广大人民群众欢迎的防治疾病的方法之一。随着我国对外政策的开放，越来越受到世界人民的信赖，它已成为世界卫生组织提出的"到2000年人人享受保健"的有效防治手段之一。它具有以下优点。

Chapter II The Advantages of Acupuncture and Moxibustion Therapy

For thousands of years acupuncture and moxibustion therapies have been widely popular as methods of preventing and treating diseases. These techniques have been increasingly acceptable by the people of the world, as the foreign policy of our country has become more open. Acupuncture and moxibustion will become one of the methods for the effective prevention and treatment of disease in support of "Health and care for all by the year 2000" statement put forward by the World Health Organization (WHO) of the United Nations.

Acupuncture and moxibustion are possessed of the following advantages.

第二章　針灸療法の利点

針灸療法は中国で、何千年以来、ずっと広範な人民大衆に喜ばれてきた疾病の預防と治療する方法の一つである。ここ数年来、中国の外交政策の開放に随って、日増しに世界各国の大勢の人人に高く評価されるにいたり、WHOが掲げられた「西歴2000年までにすべての人人に健康を」という目標を実現する効果的手段の一つであると思う。その主な利点は、次のごときものである。

（1）临床应用范围广。适应症多，疗效明显，不论是内、外、妇、儿、皮肤、五官科等，都有它的适应症，而且有些疗效明显，是单纯用中、西药物所不能比拟的。

(1) The clinical applications have a very wide range. There are many indications which show a marked response. Acupuncture and moxibustion have some indications with evidence of very high efficacy in the spheres of internal medicine, surgery, gynecology, pediatrics, dermatology, otolaryngology, ophthalmology and stomatology. There is no basis for comparison between Chinese and western medicine.

（1）臨床において、応用範囲が広い。針灸療法は適応症が多く、内科、外科、婦人科、小児科、皮膚科、五官科などいずれの分野にもその適応症があり、しかも効果が顕著で、単一の漢方薬または西洋薬を凌ぐ場合も多多ある。

（2）易学易用。针灸的学习，只要能了解基本理论，记住腧穴的部位和它的主治症，熟练操作方法，认识疾病，就可以给病人治病，学起来比较容易，用起来也较方便。当然要学精则需要下一番功夫。

(2) Simple to study and easy to use. The techniques of acupuncture and moxibustion are easy to learn and convenient to use. As long as one has knowledge of the basic therapy, remembrance of the location of points and their indications and is proficient in the manipulation, then one can treat the patient. Of course, it is advisable to make a great deal of effort for the perfection of the art.

（2）勉強しやすく、便利である。針灸治療は、その基本理論をよく学習理解し、腧穴の部位とその主治を記憶し、操作の方法に熟達し、疾病に対する認識をもてば、治療に従事することができる。したがって、勉強しやすく応用することも便利である。当然のことながら精通するには、更に努力をしなければならない。

（3）安全稳妥。在治疗中，只要注意消毒，依照针灸的操作规程进行，就不会发生任何不安全的情况，无副作用。

(3) Safe and reliable. If you ensure sterilization and proceed according to the operating rules, no hazards develop and no side-effects occur.

（3）安全で副作用がない。治療する場合、消毒に注意し、針灸の操作方法にしたがって操作すれば、危険なこともなく、副作用もない。

（4）简便经济。只要随身带上几根针和一些艾绒（或艾条）以及酒精、棉花等，随时随地就可以治病。设备简单，使用方便，同时又可以节省药费，减轻病人的经济负担。尤其用在急救时，更有其特殊的优越性。

(4) The techniques and methods are simple and economic. We can treat the disease at any time and at any place if we have some needles and moxa wool or moxa sticks, alcohol, sterilized cotton balls, and so on. Acupuncture and moxibustion may save on the costs of medicine and lighten the patient's economical burden by means of the simple equipment and convenient usage. Acupuncture and moxibustion also possess these specific advantages when used as first-aid treatments.

（4）簡便で経済的である。身の回りに針具ともぐさ及びアルコール、脱脂棉などがあれば、いつどこででも治療することができる。また設備が簡単で、便利な上に、治療費用も安く、患者にもそれ程負担をかけない。また、救急の場合には、特殊な利点がある。

第三章 针灸法

第一节 针 法

1. 针具和练习法

（1）针具：制针材料有金、银、合金等。现在多采用不锈钢针。毫针的构造分为针柄、针根、针体、针尖四个部分（图1）。

常用的毫针有多种规格，其针身的长度和直径如表1、表2。

表1 （Tab.1）

英寸/Inch	0.5	1.0	1.5	2.0	2.5	3.0	4.0	5.0
毫米/mm.	12.7	25.4	38.1	50.8	63.5	76.2	101.6	127

表2 （Tab.2）

号数/Gauge	26	28	30	32
直径 Diameter(mm.)	0.46	0.38	0.32	0.27

（2）练习法：由于毫针针体比较细软，如果没有一定的指力，很难随意进针或捻转提插。为此可先练粗短毫针，后练细长毫针。以减轻刺针时患者痛感和易于操作各种手法。

① 纸块练习法：用细软的纸，折成5×8cm大小，厚约1cm的纸块，周围用线扎紧。练习时用左手持纸块，右手拇、食、中三指持针柄，在纸块上作捻进、捻出的练习。随着指力的加强，逐渐将纸加厚（图2）。

② 棉球练习法：用棉花团成一个5～6cm直径的棉球，外用纱布扎紧。练习时，左手持棉球，右手拇、食、中三指持针，在棉球上练习提插及捻转等基本手法（图3）。

③ 自身试针：通过以上两种方法的练习，达到一定的进针指力及掌握了基本手法后，就要在自己身上试针，才能深刻地体会进针手法以及针感情况，为临床实践打好基础。

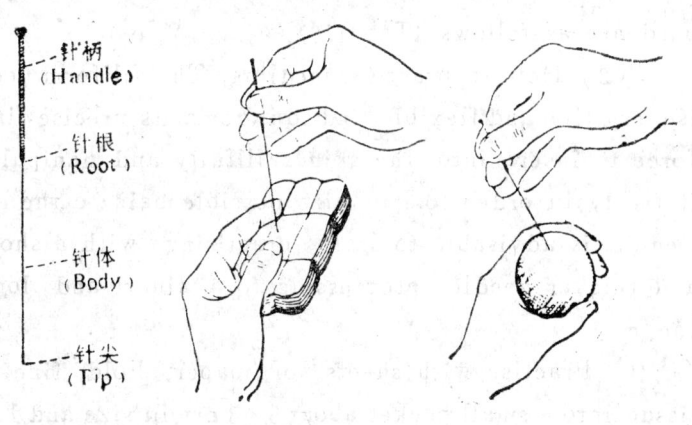

图(Fig.)1　　　图(Fig.)2　　　图(Fig.)3

Chapter III The Techniques of Acupuncture and Moxibustion

I. Manipulation of the Needle

1. The Needles and How to Use Them

(1) The Needles: The needles may be of gold, silver or alloy. The needles in most common use today are made of high quality stainless steel. On the basis of structure, the filiform needle may be divided into four parts—the handle, the root, the body and the tip (Fig.1).

The size and length of the needles most commonly used are as follows (Tab.1, 2).

(2) How to practise needling: The filiform needle is very fine and flexible, and so it demands precise finger force to insert into the skin skillfully and manipulates it freely. In order to minimize possible pain to the patient, it is advisable to start practising with a shorter and thicker needle, progressing to a finer and longer one.

① Practise with sheets of paper. Fold fine soft tissue into a small packet about 5×8 cm. in size and 1 cm. thick. Try puncturing it. Hold the paper packet in the left hand and the handle of the needle with the thumb, index and middle fingers of the right hand. Rotate the needle in and out. As your finger force grows stronger, the thickness of the packet may be increased (Fig.2).

② Practise with a small cotton cushion of about 5～6 cm. in diameter wrapped in gauze. Hold the cushion with the left hand and the needle with the thumb, index and middle fingers of the right hand. Insert the needle into it and practise the lift-thrust and rotation procedure (Fig.3).

③ Practise on your own body: This may follow the manipulation methods on paper packet and cotton cushion, so as to have personal experience of the acupuncture sensation in clinical practice.

第三章　針灸法

第一節　毫針の刺し方

1. 針具と練習法

（1）針具：針を作る材料は、金、銀、合金があるが、今はよくステンレス製の針がよく使われている。毫針の構造は（図1）のように、針柄、針根、針体、針尖の四つの部分に分けられる。

毫針の規格は多いが、よく使われている毫針の長さと直径は表1、2のようである。

（2）練習法：毫針の針体は比較的細く、柔らかいため、もし一定の指力がないと、思うままに刺しいれ、捻転提挿するこ

とがかなりむずかしい、又刺針時受針者の痛みを減軽するため、各種の手法を操作できるため、先ず指力を強める練習が必要である。練習する時、初めは短かく、ふとい針を使い、次第に細く長い針にかえてゆく。

① 重層紙練習法：薄くて柔かい紙を 5×8cm 角位の大さに切り、それを1cm位の厚さに重ねて、そのまわりを系で固く縛る。練習の際、左手で紙を持ち、右手の拇指、示指、中指で針を持って、前後に捻転し、手指に徐徐に力をいれ、捻り込み、捻り出しの練習をする。指力が強くなるにつれて、紙を次第に厚くするようにする（図2）。

② 針たんぽ練習法：棉で直径 5～6cm の棉球を作り、ガーゼでその周囲をしっかりつつむ。左手で針たんぽをつかみ、右手の拇指、示指、中指の三指で針を持ち、針たんぽで、針の上げ下げと捻りを組み合せた手法を練習する（図3）。

③ 自身で針感を経験する：上述した二種類の方法で練習し、指力が一定の強さをもつようになり、しかも基本的な手法が身についたら、更に一歩すすめ、臨床の基礎づけになるように、自分の体に針を刺し、各種の手法による反応と感覚を自身で経験する。

2．进针及出针

（1）进针：一般用右手持针，以拇、食二指捏持针柄，中指靠在食指下方贴近针根，临床上称为刺手；再以左手按押腧穴部位，临床上称为押手。两手协同动作，使针尖迅速透过皮肤，以减轻进针时的疼痛（图4）。

根据针的长短与腧穴部位的不同，所用的进针手法也各有不同，主要有以下四种：

① 指切进针：用押手拇指或食指尖按压在腧穴旁，针尖靠

近指甲刺入腧穴。此法多适用短针的进针，如刺内关、昆仑等穴（图5）。

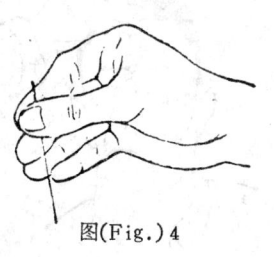

图(Fig.)4

② 骈指进针：用左手拇、食两指腹夹捏棉球，裹住针尖，直对腧穴，刺手持针柄，当押手拇、食两指下按时，刺手顺势将针刺入达一定的深度。这种方法多适用于长针的进针，如刺环跳、秩边等穴（图6）。

③ 舒张进针：用押手拇、食两指将贴近腧穴的皮肤向两侧撑开，使皮肤绷紧，易于进针。这种方法适用于皮肤松弛的部位，如腹部的天枢、关元等穴（图7）。

④ 挟持进针：用押手拇、食两指将腧穴的皮肤捏起，刺手持针从侧面刺入。这种方法多适用于肌肤较薄的部位，如刺头面部的攒竹、印堂等穴（图8）。

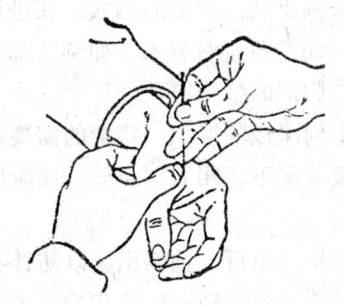

图(Fig.)5

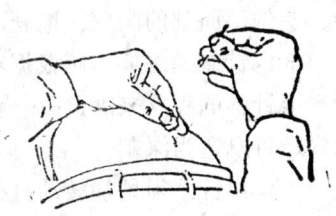

图(Fig.)6

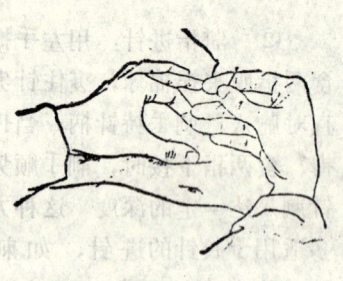
图(Fig.)7

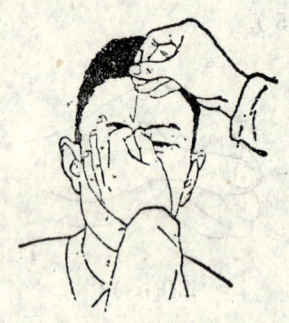
图(Fig.)8

（2）针刺的角度：根据所刺部位和治疗目的不同，针体和皮肤面的角度，可分为下列三种：

① 直刺：将针体垂直，与腧穴的皮肤面呈90度角而刺入。全身的腧穴，大多数可以直刺。

② 斜刺：某些腧穴部位，因其肌肉较薄，或腧穴深部当重要内脏所在，针刺时需使针体倾斜，一般是针体与腧穴的皮肤面呈45度角左右。如刺上肢的列缺、腹部的鸠尾，胸部的期门及背部的穴位等。

③ 横刺：又名沿皮刺。用来刺肌肤浅薄部的腧穴。在进针时，将针体与腧穴的皮肤面呈15～25度角左右刺入。如刺头部的百会、头维，面部的阳白、地仓，胸部的膻中等穴。

（3）针刺的深度：应根据不同深浅的组织、病情的需要和患者产生针感的程度来决定。一般情况下，四肢、腹部、腰骶部的腧穴，可以适当深刺。

（4）出针：须稍加转动再提出，不可一抽而出，以防针孔出血或遗留痛感。出针后根据情况酌用棉球轻轻按针孔。

2. Insertion and Withdrawal of the Needle

(1) Insertion: Generally, the needle is held with the

right hand, known clinically as the puncturing hand, with the thumb and index fingers holding the handle of the needle and the middle finger backing the index finger near the needle root. The left hand, known as the pressing hand, presses upon the area close to the point. The coordination of the two hands is conducive to a swift penetration of the needle tip into the skin, which reduces pain on insertion (Fig. 4).

According to the length of the needle and the location of the point, there are various methods of insertion. The four main techniques are as follows:

① Inserting the needle aided by the pressure of the finger of the pressing hand: Press beside the acupuncture point with the nail of the thumb or the index finger of the pressing hand, then insert the needle into the point against the nail. This method is suitable for puncturing with short needles such as those used for puncturing Neiguan, Kunlun etc. (Fig. 5).

② Inserting the needle with the help of the puncturing and pressing hands: Hold the tip of the needle wrapped in a cotton ball with the thumb and index fingers of the pressing hand; fix it directly over the selected point; meanwhile hold the handle of the needle with the puncturing hand. As the pressing hand pushes the needle tip into the skin, the puncturing hand presses it downward to the required depth. This method is suitable for puncturing with long needles, such as those used in puncturing Huantiao, Zhibian etc. (Fig. 6).

③ Inserting the needle with the fingers stretching the skin: Stretch the skin where the point is located to cause tension with the thumb and the index finger of the pressing hand to facilitate the insertion of the needle. This method is indicated for points where the skin is loose such as Tianshu, Guanyuan, etc. on the abdomen (Fig.7).

④ Inserting the needle by pinching up the skin: Pinch up the skin at the point with the thumb and index finger of the pressing hand, insert the needle into the skin sidewise with the right hand. This method is suitable for puncturing points of the head and face where the soft tissue is thin, such as Zanzhu, Yintang, etc. (Fig.8).

(2) The angle formed by the needle and the skin surface: The degree of the angles formed by the needle and the skin surface in puncturing depends upon the location of the point and the therapeutic purpose. There are three angles as following:

① Perpendicular, in which the needle is inserted perpendicularly forming a 90° angle with the skin surface. Most points on the body can be punctured perpendicularly.

② Oblique, in which the needle is inserted obliquely to form an angle of approximately 45° with the skin surface. This method is indicated for points located where the muscle is thin or close to important viscera, such as Lieque of the forearm, Jiuwei of the abdominal area, Qimen of the chest, points on the back, etc.

③ Transverse, also known as horizontal puncture when the needle enters the skin forming an angle of from 15°~25° with its surface. This method is chosen for points on the face and head where the muscle is thin, such as Baihui and Touwei of the head, Yangbai and Dicang of the face, Shanzhong of the chest, etc.

(3) Depth of needle insertion: It depends upon the thickness of the tissue where the point is located, pathological condition, and the strength of sensation the patient experiences. As a rule, points on the extremities, abdomen and lumbosacral region may be punctured deep.

(4) Withdrawal of the needle: To prevent the bleeding at the site of puncture and the after-sensation, it is necessary to rotate the needle back and forth gently before withdrawing it, then press the puncture site gently with a sterilized cotton ball upon withdrawal.

2. 進針と抜針

（1）進針：普通は右手の拇指と示指で針柄を挟み、中指は示指の下方針根に近いところにつけ、臨床では右手を刺手と称し、左手は腧穴の部位をおさえ、臨床では左手を押手と称する。針を刺す場合、両手お互いに協調させて、針先をすみやかに刺しいれ皮膚を通すようにして、患者の疼痛を軽減する（図4）。

針の長さと腧穴部位によって、進針の手法も違う。主に次の四種類ある。

① 指切式：右手の拇指と示指で針根部を持ち、左手の拇指あるいは示指の先で穴位のそばをおさえ、針先を押手の指先に近付けて、刺手の手指の圧力によって進針する。この方法は短い針を使う場合に適用する。例えば、内関、崑崙などの穴位

に用いる（図5）。

② 挾持式：左手の拇指、示指で消毒棉球を持ち、針体の下部を挾み、針先を穴位に正しく向け、右手は針柄を持ち、左手の拇指と示指で穴位に圧を加えると同時に、右手で針を押し込む。この方法は長い針を使う場合に用いる。例えば、環跳、秩辺などの穴位に刺入する場合（図6）。

③ 開き押し式：左手の拇指と示指で腧穴両側の弛んだ皮膚を広げるように緊張させて進針しやすくする。この方法は皮膚の弛んだ部位に適用する。例えば、腹部の天枢、関元などの穴位に刺入する場合（図7）。

④ 抓み押し式：左手の拇指と示指で経穴の皮膚を抓み上げ、抓み上げたところに、右手に持った針を側面から刺入する。この方法は顔面部のような筋肉の浅い部位に用いられる。例えば、顔面部の攢竹、印堂などの穴位に適用する（図8）。

（2）針の刺入角度：針を刺入する部位と治療の目的が違うことにより、針と皮膚表面の角度が三種類に分けられる。

① 直刺：針体を垂直にして、針と腧穴の皮膚表面との角度を90度にして刺入する。この刺入法は全身の大多数の腧穴に使われる。

② 斜刺：一部の腧穴の部位では、筋肉が薄く、または深部に重要な内臓があるので、刺入する場合には、針体を傾斜させ、針体と腧穴部位の皮膚表面との角度を45度位にして刺入する。例えば、上肢の列缺、腹部の鳩尾、胸部の期門及び背部の穴位などに適用する。

③ 横刺：沿皮刺ともいう。筋肉のあさいところの腧穴に用いる。針を刺す時、針体を経穴の皮膚との角度を15〜25度位にして刺入する。例えば頭部の百会、頭維、顔面部の陽白、地倉、胸部の膻中などの経穴を用いる場合。

（3）針刺の深さ：筋肉組織の厚き、症状と患者の針感に

よって決められる。普通は、四肢、腹部、腰仙部などの部位にある腧穴は適当に深刺できる。

（4）抜針：抜針した後の出血と後遺疼痛感を防ぐため、急激な，または乱暴な抜針をしてはいけない、ゆっくり捻りながら抜き出す。針を抜きだした後、時には棉球で軽く腧穴を按摩する必要がある。

3．注意事项

（1）过饥、过饱、酒醉、过劳时或身体虚弱的患者，应注意少针或缓针。

（2）妊娠3个月以下者，少腹部、腰骶部穴位禁针；3个月以上者，上腹部、腰骶部以及其他一些能引起剧烈针感的腧穴，如合谷、三阴交、昆仑、至阴等均禁针。婴儿的囟门部位禁针。

3. Precaution

(1) It is advisable to apply few needles or to delay giving acupuncture treatment for patients who are famished, over-eaten, tipsy, over fatigued or very weak.

(2) It is contraindicated to puncture points on the lower abdomen and lumbosacral region for women pregnant under three months. After three months of pregnancy it is also contraindicated to puncture the points of the upper abdomen, and those causing strong sensation such as Hegu, Sanyinjiao, Kunlun and Zhiyin. The fontanelle of infants should not be punctured.

3．注意事項

（1）空腹時、食べすぎ、飲酒時、疲れすぎあるいは、体力虚弱などの患者に、針の数をすくなくにするか、あるいは、弱刺激をあたえること。

（2）3个月に未たない妊婦の下腹部、腰仙部の穴位には、針は禁忌である。3个月以上の妊婦の上腹部、腰仙部及びはげしい針感を起させる腧穴、例えば合谷、三陰交、崑崙、至陰なども同じく禁忌である、赤子の泉門の部位に針を刺してはいけない。

4．异常现象的处理

（1）晕针：由于患者体质虚弱，或初次接受针刺而精神紧张，或针刺手法过重等原因，可有晕针现象的发生。晕针的先兆，多出现头晕目眩、心烦欲呕，继而面色苍白、目呆、神滞；严重的可有昏厥，人事不省，脉搏沉伏等虚脱症状。医者在发现晕针先兆时，应立即出针安慰患者，嘱其躺卧，轻者给些热开水，休息片刻即可恢复；重者用指掐或针刺人中、中冲等穴，再灸百会、足三里，促使苏醒。如仍不解除时，应采取其他急救措施。

（2）滞针：针刺入后，针下异常紧涩，不能作捻转和提插动作的叫滞针。遇有这种情况，应根据不同原因进行处理：

因肌肉一时性紧张所致的，应留针一段时间，然后再行捻转，即可出针。或在所刺腧穴的周围按压或针刺，以缓解局部紧张状态而顺利出针。

因针体受肌纤维缠绕而不能退出时，应轻轻捻转，将缠绕的肌纤维回释，再行轻度提插，等待松弛后，便可退出。

（3）弯针：由于进针时指力不匀、用力过猛，或针下碰到坚硬的组织以及患者在针刺入后移动了体位，或针柄受到外物碰

撞等，均可使针体弯曲。如系轻度的弯曲，可慢慢地将针提出，不能再行捻转；弯曲的角度过大时，应顺前弯的方向轻轻捻动，向针柄倾斜的方向慢慢退出。如果由于体位移动所造成的，应先矫正体位，再行退针。

（4）折针：由于进针后强力捻转，肌肉挛急，或体位移动，尤其是针的材料不纯，针根剥蚀，或针根损伤，都可能造成折针。如遇到这种现象，医者要沉着，嘱咐患者不要移动体位。如果针体尚露在体表外面，用镊子取出；如针体已陷入深部，便须经手术取出。因此在临床上必须注意，仔细检查针的质量，并在选针时要注意针身的长度比准备刺入的深度长，以防止折针事故发生。

（5）血肿：出针后，如针孔处有红色小点，这是临床上常见的现象，不须处理，自行消失。如出针后皮肤呈青紫色或肿起，这是误伤血管所致，宜按摩局部以后用热敷，帮助消散。

（6）后遗感：在出针后，局部遗留酸痛不适的感觉，多系针刺手法过重所致。轻者以手在局部上下循按，即可消失；较重的除循按外，并在局部施灸，也可很快的消除。

4. Management of Possible Accidents in Acupuncture

(1) Fainting: This may occur due to weakness or to nervous tension on receiving acupuncture for the first time, or to too forceful manipulation. The prodromes are dizziness and vertigo, irritability, nausea, pallor, staring eyes and dull appearance. In severe cases there may be shock and unconsiousness with a deep pulse. The needles should be removed at once and help the patient to lie down for relaxing. In mild cases, the symptoms will disappear after a short rest or taking some warm dranks. In severe cases, press Renzhong with the fingernail, or

puncture Renzhong and Zhongchong. Moxibustion may be applied to Baihui and Zusanli. Generally the patient will respond, but if not, then other emergency measures should be taken.

(2) Stuck Needle: After the needle is inserted it is found at times difficult or impossible to rotate, lift and thrust. This situation is known as stuck needle, due to various causes.

If it is due to muscle spasm, the needle should be retained for a while, and then rotated for removal. Another method is to press the area around the needle, or puncture another point nearby, to relieve the muscle tension.

If the needle is entangled with fibrous tissue, rotate it gently and slowly to disentangle it. Lift and thrust slightly until the muscle is completely relaxed, then withdraw the needle.

(3) Bent Needle: This generally happens when the needle is inserted more forcefully with uneven finger force or too forcefully, or the needle strikes hard tissue. The handle of the needle may be struck accidentally, or the patient may suddenly change position while the needle is in place. If the bend is slight, the needle may be removed slowly without rotating. If pronounced, move the needle slightly and withdraw it by following the course of the bend. If the patient has changed position, move him to his original position and then withdraw the needle.

(4) Broken Needle: Forceful manipulation of the needle, muscle spasm, changing position of the patient,

or poor quality of the needle or eroded base of needle all may be the causes. The doctor should be calm and advise the patient not to move. If the broken needle protrudes above the skin, remove it with forceps. If it is completely under the skin, surgery will be necessary. To prevent accidents, careful inspection of the quality of the needle should be made clinically. The needle must be somewhat longer than the required depth of the insertion.

(5) Hematoma: After withdrawal of the needle, a pin-point red mark may remain. This is considered normal, and it will disappear of its own accord. If a bruise or swelling occurs due to injury to vessels, the site should be massaged and hot compresses applied to promote absorption of the blood.

(6) After withdrawal of the needle, there may remain an uncomfortable feeling due to over-stimulation. If the sensation is not too severe, it may be relieved by gently massaging the local area. If the discomfort persists, it may be relieved by applying moxibustion.

4. 針刺時に生じた異常の処理

（1）暈針：患者の体質が虚弱、あるいは未経験者、精神緊張、または、針刺手法が強すぎるなどにより、暈針が引き起されうる。暈針が現れる場合、患者は、めまい、胸部苦悶感、悪心を訴え、顔色蒼白、目呆、精神異常となり、重症では、脈搏微弱、意識消失、昏迷などショックの症状が見られる。医者が暈針の前兆を発見した時は、直ちに抜針して、患者を寝かせる。軽い場合は、熱いお湯を飲ませ、しばらく安静にしていれ

ば、回復する。重い場合は、医者は爪甲で、人中穴を押えつけるか、人中、中衝などの穴位を針刺する。さらに、百会、足三里にお灸をして、意識を回復させる。もし以上の措置を施しても、症状が改善されない場合には、他の救急手当法を取るべきである。

　（2）滯針：刺針部に、非常に緊張した渋滯感があり、提挿、捻転ができなくなるのを滯針という。臨床では、その原因によって次のような措置を施す。

　筋肉の一時的緊張によるものは、しばらく置針して、捻転すれば、抜針することができる。あるいは経穴の周囲を指圧するか、またはもう一本針を刺すと、筋肉が弛緩して、抜針することができる。

　針体に組織繊維がまとわりついた事が原因の場合には、針を逆の方向に軽く回し、すこし提挿し、針が動くようになってから抜針する。

　（3）彎針：針刺する時、力が強すぎ、指力の不均衡、あるいは針尖がかたい組織にぶつかったり、または、針刺した後、患者が体を動かし体位が変ったり、外物が針柄に触れたりなどの時に、彎針を引き起しやすい。針体の彎曲が小さい場合は、針を捻転しないようにゆっくり抜き出す。彎曲が大きい場合は静かに針体を揺り動かし、針柄がどの方向に曲っているかを調べ、その方向に沿って抜き出す。患者が体位を変えたことが原因の場合は、まずもとの体位にもどしてから、抜針する。

　（4）折針：針を刺した後、捻針する時に力をいれすぎて、筋肉が強く収縮し、あるいは病人が体位を変たりした場合、あるいは針体の腐蝕、針根の損傷、針の材質不良等、これ等が原因となり、折針を引き起しやすい。折針を発見したら、医者は冷静にかまえ、患者にはもとの体位を保持させ、決してあわててはならない。折れた針体が皮膚の外に現われている場合

は、ピンセットで抜き取る。深部で折れ、折端が全然外部に現われていない時は、手術によって取り出す。折針を防止するためには、針刺する前に針具をこまかく検査し、前述の折針の原因を作らないこと、針の長さは刺入する深さより長いのを選ぶことに注意しなければならない。

　　（5）血腫：抜針した後、針刺した部位に小さな赤い斑点ができることがあるが、これは臨床でよく見られる現象で、普通は手当をしなくても自然に消えてしまう。もし局所が青く、かなり腫れた場合は、血管を傷つけたためで、按摩あるいは温湿布で消散させる。

　　（6）後遺感：抜針した後、局所にだるい、痛みなどいやな感じが残ることは、多くは針刺手法が強すぎたためである。軽い場合は局所をもめば消失する。重い場合は、局所をもむほかに、局部にお灸をすれば、比較的速く消失する。

第二节　灸　法

灸法是以艾绒为主要原料所做成的艾炷或艾条，燃烧后熏灼穴位以达到防治疾病的一种方法。

艾绒是用艾叶（菊科植物）的叶片，经过晒干研细，去掉粗梗杂质，成为柔软的纤维。它具有温通经络、祛除寒湿、促进人体机能旺盛的作用。艾炷是将艾绒少许置于平板上，以拇、食、中三指捏成上尖下宽的圆锥形。如麦粒大、枣核大或拇指大。艾条是用桑皮纸将艾绒卷成一定大小的烟卷状，用于熏灼，较艾炷为简便。

临床常用的灸治方法，可分为艾炷灸、艾条灸及温针灸三类（图9、10、11、12）。

— 25 —

II. Moxibustion

Moxibustion treats and prevents diseases by applying heat to points or certain locations of the human body. The material used is mainly "moxa-wool" in the form of a large cigarette or a small cone.

Moxa-wool is made of dry moxa, or mugwort leaves (Artemisia vulgaris), ground finely, with the coarse stems removed. It has the properties of warming and removing obstruction of the channels, eliminating cold and damp and thus promoting normal function of the organs. Moxa cones are made by placing a small amount of moxa wool on a board and kneading it into a cone with the thumb, index and middle fingers. The size may be similar to that of a grain of wheat; the size of a date stone, or the size of the upper part of the thumb. Moxa sticks are much more convenient to use than moxa cones. Moxa sticks are made by simply rolling moxa wool into the shape of a large paper cigarette made of mulberry bark. They are easier than moxa cones for applying heat to points.

Clinically, there are three methods of application; i.e. with moxa cones, with moxa sticks, and with warming needles (Fig. 9, 10, 11, 12).

第二節 灸法

灸法はもぐさで艾柱あるいは艾条を作り、それに点火し

て、人体の一定部位を刺激することにより、疾病を治療する方法である。

　艾はよもぎ（菊科植物）の葉をつみとり、乾燥させた後、こまかくし、さらに雑質を取り除くと、柔かい繊維のような艾になる。艾は経脈を温通し、寒湿を取り除き、人体の機能を旺盛にする作用がある。したがって、艾をお灸の材料としたことは、意味がある訳である。艾柱は、少量のもぐさを平板におき、拇指、示指、中指でひねり、上が小さく、下が大きい円錐体にして、麦の粒、ナツメの核、あるいは拇指先の大きさなどの三種にする。艾条は桑皮紙で艾を包み、適当な太さのたばこのような棒状につくる。その一端に点火して、患部を薫する。操作方法は艾柱より簡単である。臨床では、艾柱灸、艾条灸及び温針灸など三種類に分けられる（図9、10、11、12）。

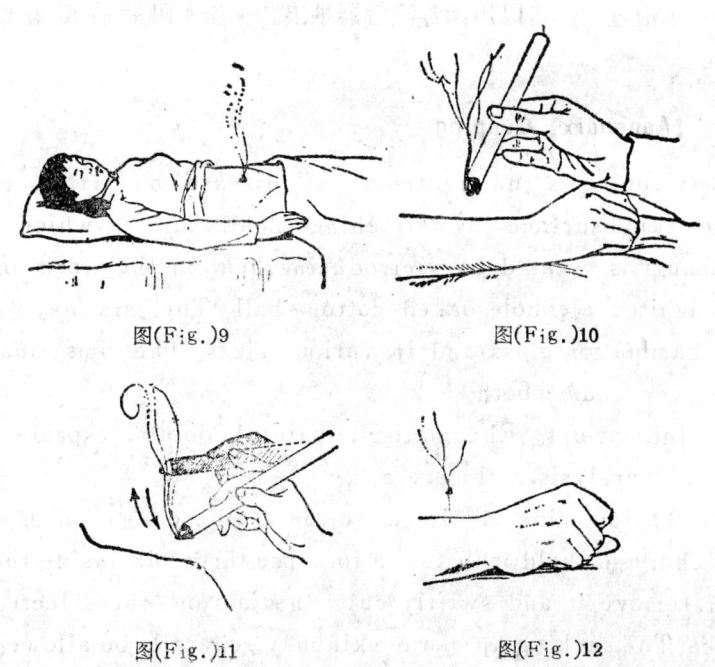

図(Fig.)9　　　　　　図(Fig.)10

図(Fig.)11　　　　　　図(Fig.)12

【附】拔罐疗法

用罐口光滑平整大小不等的竹罐、玻璃火罐，通过酒精棉球等的燃烧，使罐内出现较高的温度而形成负压吸附于皮肤表面，以治疗疾病的一种方法。

适应范围：多用于痹痛、扭伤、口眼歪斜、哮喘等。

操作方法：用长镊子夹住蘸有95%酒精的棉球，点燃后送入罐内，立即抽出，迅速地将罐口按在需要拔罐的部位。一般病证拔10～15分钟，然后右手持罐，左手用指压在罐口傍侧皮肤，使空气进入罐内，即可起罐。

注意事项：高热抽搐、皮肤过敏、水肿、有出血倾向者，以及孕妇腹部均不宜应用。拔罐后局部皮肤有青紫郁血现象，一般几天后即消失。如皮肤上有小水泡，几天后也能吸收，故不需处理。水泡过大，可以用消毒注射器抽出。再涂龙胆紫后覆盖敷料。

【Appendix】 Cupping

Cupping is the treatment of disease by suction to the skin surface by attaching small jars in which a vacuum is created by introducing heat in the form of an ignited alcohol-soaked cotton ball. The jars may be of bamboo or glass and in various sizes. The rims must be even and smooth.

Indications: Rheumatism, painful joints, sprains, facial paralysis, asthma, etc.

Manipulation: Ignite a cotton ball soaked in 95% alcohol and hold it between forceps, thrust it inside the jar, remove it and swiftly cup the jar on the selected area. The sucking up of the skin may generally be allowed to go on for 10~15 minutes. To remove, let air into the jar by holding it in the right hand and pressing the skin at the rim of the jar with the left.

Precautions: It is not advisable to apply cupping to patients with high fever, convulsions, allergic skin diseases, edema, or hemorrhagic tendencies, or to the abdominal area of women during pregnancy. The local area will show blood congestion after cupping, the bruise on the skin surface be gradually disappeared within a few days. If minute blisters form, they may also be absorbed after one or two days. However for any large blisters, it is advisable to drain the fluid with a sterilized syringe, and apply gentian violet before dressing.

【附】抜罐療法

切口が滑らかで平らな、大きさの異る竹罐、ガラス罐等を器具とする。アルコール棉球を燃やして、罐内の温度を高くし、マイナス圧を生じさせることによって、皮膚に吸着させ、疾病を治療する方法である。

適応範囲: 痺痛、軟部組織の損傷、口と目の歪み、喘息などによく用いられる。

操作方法: アルコール棉球を長めのピンセットで挾み、それに点火し、罐内でしばらく燃やしてから取り出し、すばやく罐を治療すべき部位にかぶせて吸着させる。一般の病症には、10~15分間施す、罐をはずす時は、右手で罐を持ち、左手で罐の周囲の皮膚を押えると、罐内に空気が入り、罐はすぐはずれる。

注意事項: 高熱による搔搔、皮膚過敏、水腫あるいは出血傾向のある患者及び妊婦の腹部などは避けるべきである。抜罐

した後、局所の皮膚が赤紫になり瘀血現象が見られるが、普通は数日後に消失する。小さい水泡ができても、数日で吸収され、特別の処置をする必要はない。水泡がかなり大きい場合は、消毒した注射器で、水泡内の水を吸え出した後、ゲンチアナバイオレットを塗り、消毒ガーゼをかけておけばよい。

第四章 经络与腧穴

第一节 分类及分布

经络主要包括十二经脉、奇经八脉和十五络脉等。十二经脉和奇经八脉中的督脉和任脉，合称十四经脉，其上各有专穴，与针灸临床的关系最为密切。十二经对称地分布于人体的两侧，其中手三阴经从胸走向手，手三阳经从手走向头，足三阳经从头走向足，足三阴经从足走向腹、胸。任脉和督脉均出于会阴，分别向上行于人体前后正中线。

腧穴一般分为十四经腧穴，经外奇穴和阿是穴三类。十四经腧穴是指属于十四经系统的腧穴，是全身腧穴的主要部分，共计361穴。其中十二经脉的腧穴为左右对称的双穴，督脉和任脉的腧穴则分别分布于前后正中线的单穴。经外奇穴是指有固定位置而尚未归入十四经系统的经验有效穴。阿是穴是指根据病证的压痛点或其他病理反应点来定位的一些腧穴，它没有固定的位置和穴名，即"以痛为腧"。

Chapter IV Channels, Collaterals and Points

I. Classification and Distribution

The system of channels and collaterals mainly consists of the twelve regular channels, the eight extra channels and the fifteen collaterals. The twelve regular channels, together with the Ren Channel and the Du Channel of the eight extra channels, form the fourteen channels. There are points for applying acupuncture and moxibustion along each channel. The twelve regular channels are distributed symmetrically on the right and left sides of the body. Among them, the three yin channels of the hand run from the chest to the hand, the three yang channels of the hand from the hand to the head, the three yang channels of the foot from the head to the foot, and the three yin channels of the foot from the foot to the abdomen and chest. The Ren and Du Channels originate from the perineum and ascend along the anterior and the posterior midline of the body respectively.

Points are classified into 3 categories: points of the 14 channels, extraordinary points and Ahshi points. The points of the 14 channels, which make up the majority of all the points on the human body, are 361 in number. Those of the 12 regular channels exist in pairs distributed symmetrically on the left and the right side of the body, while those of the Ren and Du Channels are single, aligning on the anterior and the posterior midline respectively. Extraordinary points are useful in therapy, though discovered in the course of practice. They have definite locations but are not listed in the system of the 14 channels.

Ahshi points are tender spots or sensitive spots present in certain diseases. They have neither definite locations nor names, that is, "Where there is a painful spot, there is an acupuncture point".

第四章　経絡と腧穴

第一節　分類及び分布

経絡には主に十二経脈、奇経八脈と十五絡脈などが含まれている。十二経脈と奇経八脈の督脈と任脈をあわせて十四経脈という。十四経脈には決まっている穴位があり、針灸の臨床にもっとも密接な関係をもつものである。十二の経絡は、人体の両側に対称的に分布している、そのうち手の三陰経は、胸部から上肢へ、手の三陽経は、上肢から頭部へ、足の三陽経は、頭から下肢へ、足の三陰経は、足から腹部、胸部へ走行する。任脈と督脈は、会陰部から出て、それぞれ人体の前後正中線を上行する。

腧穴は、十四経腧穴、経外奇穴、阿是穴など三種類に分け

られる。十四経腧穴は、十四経系に属するツボを指し、全身腧穴の主なものであり、あわせて361穴ある。十二経脈の腧穴は、左右対称的に配列している双穴であり、督脈と任脈の腧穴は前後正中線に配列している単穴である。経外奇穴は、位置が明確で、治療効果も著しいが、十四経に帰属していない経験穴を指す。阿是穴は、病的な圧痛点、あるいは反応点等によって決定されたツボを指す。したがって、阿是穴というのは、一定した部位ではなく、当然穴名もなく、即ち「痛むところを腧とする」というものである。

第二节 腧穴的定位法

腧穴各有一定位置。腧穴定位是否准确，会直接影响到治疗效果。要做到定位准确，就必须掌握一定的定位方法。临床常用的定位方法有三种：

1. 解剖标志法 人体体表有各种解剖标志，可作为定位的主要依据。如骨节、肌肉的隆起或凹陷、皮肤的皱纹、发际、爪甲、乳头、脐、眼、唇等，在这些标志附近的腧穴，就可以直接根据标志来定位。

II. Methods for Locating Points

Each point has a definite location which must be determined accurately for effective therapeutic result. The following three methods for locating points accurately have been introduced.

1. According to Anatomical Landmarks Anatomical landmarks on the body surface, such as prominence or depression of the bone, joint, tendon, muscle, skin crease, hairline, border of nail, nipple, umbilicus, eye and mouth, are of specific significance in locating points. If the sites of points are in the vicinity of or on such landmarks, they can be located directly.

第二節　腧穴の定位法

腧穴は一定の位置にあり、臨床に臨んで取穴した腧穴の位置が正確か否かは、直接治療の効果に影響してくる。正しく腧穴の部位を決めるためには、必ず一定の定位法をマスターしなければならない。常用される定位法には次の三種類がある。

1. 解剖標志法　人体の体表にある各種の解剖学的要素を定位の主な根拠とする。例えば関節、筋肉の突起と陥凹、皮膚の皺、髪の生際、爪甲、乳頭、臍および目、口唇などを基準として、その近くにある腧穴の位置が定められる。

2. 骨度分寸法　在体表解剖标志的基础上，离开这些标志较远的腧穴，则采用一种折量的方法——骨度分寸法。这种方法是将人体不同部位的长度或宽度，分别规定为一定等分（每一等分称为1寸），作为量取腧穴的标准。

（1）头部

直寸：前发际至后发际折作12寸。

前发际不明者，可从眉心上行加3寸；后发际不明者，可从大椎上行加3寸，即眉心至大椎之间折作18寸。

横寸：耳后两乳突之间折作9寸，两头维之间折作9寸。

（2）胸腹部

直寸：胸部以肋间隙为根据。侧胸部腋纹头至11肋骨端折作12寸。上腹部，胸肋角至脐中折作8寸。下腹部，脐中至耻骨联

合上缘折作5寸。

横寸：两乳头或两锁骨中线之间均折作8寸。

（3）背部

直寸：以脊椎棘突为根据。

横寸：肩胛骨内侧缘至脊柱正中线之间折作3寸。

（4）上肢部

上臂：腋纹头至肘横纹折作9寸。

前臂：肘横纹至腕横纹折作12寸。

（5）下肢部

大腿内侧，从平耻骨联合上缘至股骨内上髁折作18寸；外侧，从股骨大转子隆起处至膝中折作19寸。

小腿内侧，从胫骨内髁下缘至内踝高点，折作13寸；外侧，从膝中至外踝高点折作16寸（图13）。

2. **Proportional Measurement** On the basis of anatomical landmarks, a measuring method has been established for locating points at a distance from anatomical landmarks — proportional measurement. The width or length of various portions of the human body are divided respectively into definite numbers of equal divisions, each division being termed one cun (寸). These are taken as the unit of measurement in locating points.

(1) Head

Longitudinal measurement: The distance from the anterior hairline to the posterior hairline is taken as 12 cun. If the anterior hairline is indistinguishable, measurement can be taken from the glabella and 3 cun added. If the posterior hairline is also indistinguishable, measurement can be taken from point Dazhui, and 3 cun added. The distance from the glabella to Dazhui then is 18 cun.

Transverse measurement: The distance between the two mastoid processes is 9 cun, as is that between points Touwei of both sides.

(2) Chest and abdomen

Longitudinal measurement: Measurement of the chest is based on the intercostal spaces. The distance from the end of the axillary fold on the lateral side of the chest to the tip of the 11th rib is measured as 12 cun. On the upper abdomen, the distance from the sternocostal angle to the centre of the umbilicus is measured as 8 cun. On the lower abdomen, the distance between the centre of the umbilicus and the upper border of symphysis pubis is 5 cun.

Transverse measurement: The distance between the two nipples or the two midclavicular lines is 8 cun.

(3) Back

Longitudinal measurement: This is based on the spinous processes of the vertebral column.

Transverse measurement: The distance between the medial border of the scapula and the posterior midline is 3 cun.

(4) Upper extremities

Upper arm: The distance between the end of the axillary fold and the transverse cubital crease is 9 cun.

Forearm: The distance between the transverse cubital crease and the transverse carpal crease is 12 cun.

(5) Lower extremities

The medial aspect of the thigh: The distance from the level of the upper border of symphysis pubis to the medial epicondyle of femur is 18 cun.

The lateral aspect of the thigh: The distance from the prominence of great trochanter to the middle of patella is 19 cun.

The medial aspect of the leg: The distance from the lower border of the medial condyle of tibia to the tip of the medial malleolus is 13 cun.

The lateral aspect of the leg: The distance between the centre of patella and the tip of the lateral malleolus is 16 cun (Fig.13).

2. 骨度分寸法　解剖学的標記法に基づいて、その標記より割合に遠く離れた部位にある腧穴を表わす場合は、折量法即ち骨度分寸法を用いる。人体の各部のそれぞれの長さあるいは幅をいくつかに等分し、それを基準とする方法である。これは患者自身の一定部位を寸法の根拠とするため、肥瘦、長短に関係なく、どの人にも適用する。よく使われている骨度分寸法は次のようなものである。

（1）頭部

直寸：前頭部の髪の生際から、後頭部の髪の生際までを12寸とする。

前頭部の髪の生際のはっきりしない人は眉間中央の上3寸の所を基準とする。後頭部の髪の生際がはっきりしない場合は、大椎穴の上3寸の所を基準とする。即ち、眉間中央から大椎穴までは18寸となる。

横寸：耳後の両乳様突起の間を9寸とし、両側頭維穴の間を9寸とする。

（2）胸腹部

直寸：胸部は、肋間を測る尺度とし、腋窩横紋から第11肋骨までを12寸とする。上腹部では、胸骨剣状突起から臍までを8寸とする。下腹では、臍から恥骨結合の上縁までを5寸とする。

横寸：両乳頭あるいは両鎖骨中央間を8寸とする。

（3）背部

直寸：脊椎の棘突起を取穴の基準とする。

横寸：肩胛骨の脊柱縁から背部正中線までを3寸とする。

（4）上肢部

上腕：腋の横紋の前端から肘の横紋までを9寸とする。

前腕：肘の横紋から腕の横紋までを12寸とする。

（5）下肢部

大腿内側：恥骨結合の上縁から大腿骨内側上髁までを18寸とする。

外側は、大腿骨の大転子から膝窩横紋までを19寸とする。

下腿内側、脛骨の内側髁の下縁から内踝までを13寸とする。外側は膝蓋骨の下縁から外踝までを16寸とする（図13）。

3．手指比量法　这是以患者手指的长度与宽度为标准来量取腧穴的一种方法。较常用的，一种是以中指屈曲时，当第二指节两端横纹头之间的距离作为1寸（称为同身寸），另一种是以食、中、无名、小指并拢，于中指一、二指关节背侧横纹处相平，四个手指的宽度作为3寸（称为一夫指）。这种方法可在骨度分寸的基础上参考应用（图14、15）。

3. **Finger Measurement**　The length and breadth of the patient's finger(s) are used as a criterion for

— 38 —

locating points. The commonly used measuring methods are as follows:

When the middle finger is flexed, the distance between the two ends of the creases of the interphalangeal joints is taken as one cun (measuring with the middle finger).

The breadth of the four fingers (index, middle, ring and little fingers) close together at the level of the skin crease of the proximal interphalangeal joint at the dorsum of the middle finger is taken as 3 cun (measuring with the four fingers) (Fig. 14, 15).

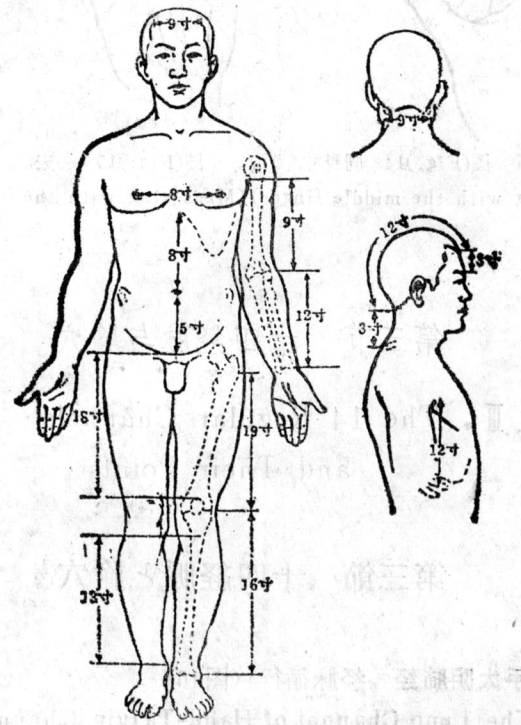

图(Fig.) 13 骨度分寸示意图 (Proportional unit)

3. 指寸法 患者自身の指の長さと幅を測定するための基準として、穴を取る方法である。よく使用されている方法は、患者自身の中指と親指で輪を作り、中指の第一、第二関節にできた横紋間の距離を1寸とする（同身寸という）。あるいは、示指、中指、薬指、小指を合せて、四横指とし、四横指の第二関節の幅を3寸とする（一夫指という）。この方法は、骨度分寸法を基にして、参考的に応用する（図14、15）。

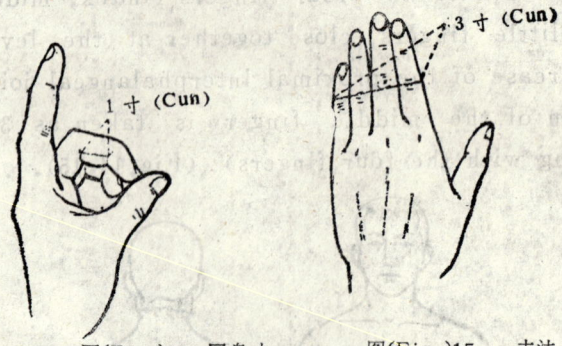

図(Fig.)14 同身寸　　　図(Fig.)15 一夫法
(Measuring with the middle finger)(Measuring with the four fingers)

第三节　十四经脉与腧穴

III. The 14 Regular Channels and Their Points

第三節　十四経脈と腧穴

1. 手太阴肺经 经脉循行（图16）。
The Lung Channel of Hand-Taiyin Channel Course

(Fig.16).

手の太陰肺経 その経脈の循行は(図16)のようである。

列 缺

【位置】在前臂茎突的上方，腕横纹上1.5寸。两手虎口交叉时 一手之食指押在另一手的腕后桡骨茎突上，当食指尖所指

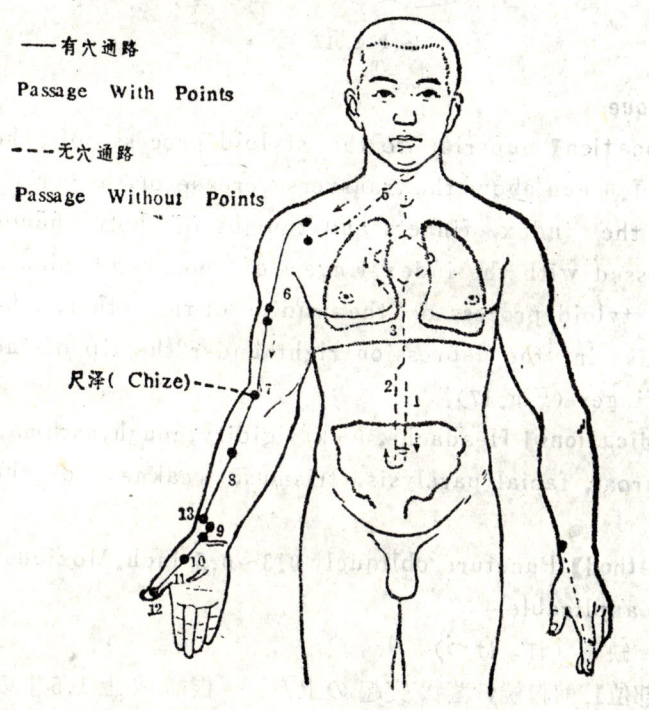

―― 有穴通路
Passage With Points

---- 无穴通路
Passage Without Points

尺泽(Chize)

图(Fig.)16 手太阴肺经循行示意图(The Lung Channel of Hand-Taiyin)

— 41 —

处是穴（图17）。

【主治】头痛项强，咳嗽，气喘，咽喉肿痛，口眼歪斜，牙关紧闭，手腕无力。

【刺灸法】斜刺0.3～0.5寸；可灸。

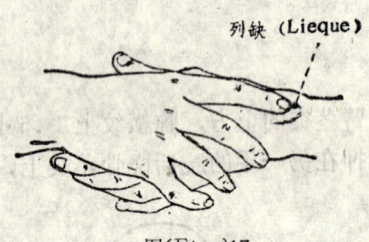

图(Fig.)17

Lieque

【Location】 Superior to the styloid process of the radius, 1.5 cun above the transverse crease of the wrist. When the index fingers and thumbs of both hands are crossed with the index finger of one hand placed on the styloid process of the radius of the other, the point is in the depression right under the tip of the index finger (Fig.17).

【Indications】 Headache, neck rigidity, cough, asthma, sore throat, facial paralysis, trismus, weakness of the wrist.

【Method】 Puncture obliquely 0.3～0.5 inch. Moxibustion is applicable.

列　缺　（れっけつ）

【部位】前膊橈骨茎状突起の上方、手根横紋上1.5寸のところ。両手の母指と示指を交叉して、橈骨茎状突起の上で示指先のあたるところ（図17）。

【主治】頭痛、頭項部強直（肌肉、筋脈が引っぱられる症

状)、咳、喘息、咽喉腫痛、口と目の歪み、口噤（歯をくいしばる)、手首無力。

【刺灸法】0.3～0.5寸斜刺し、灸ができる。

太　渊

【位置】在掌后横纹上，桡动脉桡侧凹陷中（图18）。
【主治】气喘，咳嗽，咳血，咽喉肿痛，胸痛，心悸，前臂内侧痛。
【刺灸法】直刺0.2～0.3寸；可灸。
Taiyuan
【Location】At the transverse crease of the wrist, in the depression on the radial side of the radial artery (Fig.18).
【Indications】Asthma, cough, hemoptysis, sore throat, palpitation, pain in the chest and the medial aspect of the forearm.
【Method】Puncture perpendicularly 0.2～0.3 inch. Moxibustion is applicable.

太　渊　（たいえん）

【部位】内側手関節横紋、橈骨動脈の橈側陷凹部（図18）。
【主治】喘息、咳、喀血、咽喉腫痛、胸痛、心悸、前腕内側痛。
【刺灸法】0.2～0.3寸直刺し、灸ができる。

鱼　际

【位置】在第1掌骨中点之桡侧，赤白肉际（图18）。

— 43 —

【主治】咳嗽，咳血，咽喉肿痛，发热。
【刺灸法】直刺0.5～0.7寸；可灸。

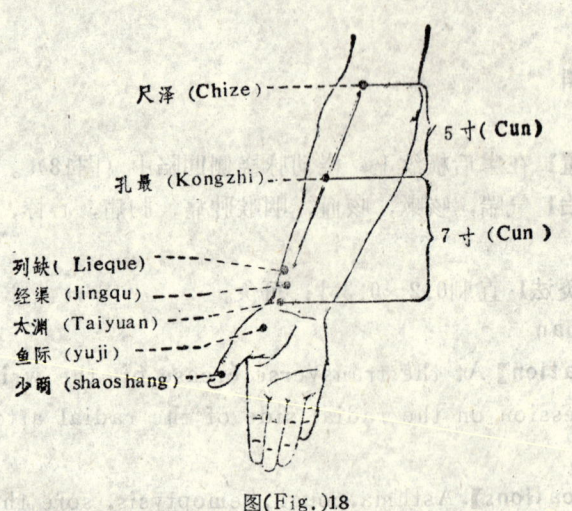

图(Fig.)18

Yuji

【Location】On the radial aspect of the midpoint of the 1st metacarpal bone, on the junction of the red and white skin (i.e., the junction of the dorsum and palm of the hand)(Fig.18).

【Indications】Cough, hemoptysis, sore throat, fever.

【Method】Puncture perpendicularly 0.5～0.7 inch. Moxibustion is applicable.

魚際　　　　　（ぎょさい）

【部位】第一中手骨の中点の橈側、赤白皮膚の肌目にとる（図18）。

【主治】咳、喀血、咽喉腫痛、発熱。

【刺灸法】0.5～0.7寸直刺し、灸ができる。

少　商

【位置】拇指桡侧指甲角后1分许（图18）。
【主治】咳嗽，气喘，咽喉肿痛，鼻衄，手指挛痛，热病，昏厥，癫狂。
【刺灸法】向上斜刺0.1寸或三棱针点刺出血。
Shaoshang
【Location】On the radial side of the thumb, about 0.1 cun posterior to the corner of the nail (Fig.18).
【Indications】Cough, asthma, sore throat, epistaxis, contracture and pain of fingers, febrile diseases, loss of consciousness, mental disorders.
【Method】Puncture obliquely upward 0.1 inch, or prick with three-edged needle to cause bleeding.
少　商　（しょうしょう）
【部位】拇指の橈側、爪甲角より0.1寸後方（図18）。
【主治】咳、喘息、咽喉腫痛、鼻血、指の痙攣痛、熱性病、昏睡、癲癇。
【刺灸法】上に向け0.1寸斜刺し、或は三棱針で瀉血する。

2. 手阳明大肠经　经脉循行（图19）。
The Large Intestine Channel of Hand-Yangming Channel Course (Fig.19).

手の陽明大腸経 その経脈の循行は（図19）のようである。

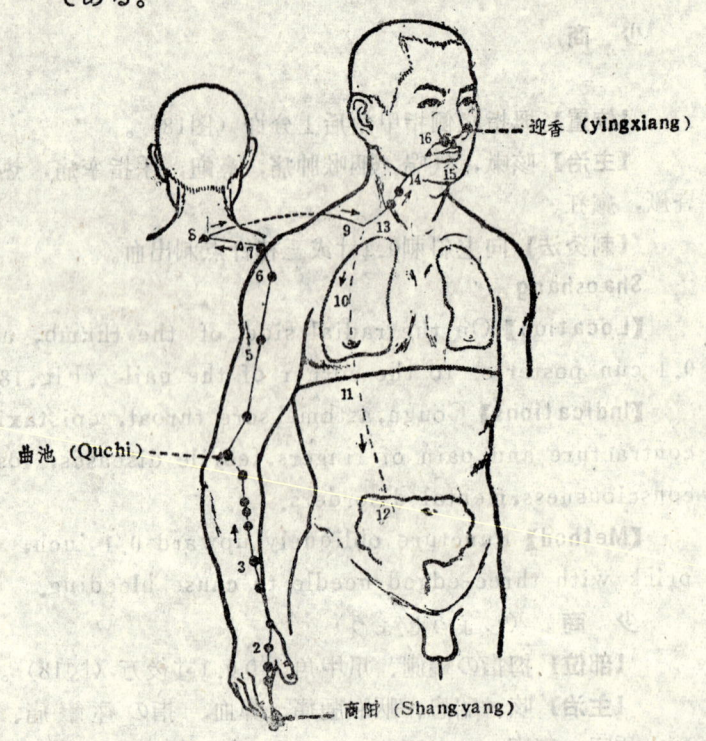

図(Fig.)19 手阳明大肠经循行示意图
(The Large Intestine Channel of Hand-Yangming)

商 阳

【位置】食指桡側指甲角后1分许（图19）。

【主治】齿痛，咽喉肿痛，颌肿，手指麻木，热病，昏厥。

【刺灸法】斜刺0.1寸，三棱针点刺出血。

Shangyang

【Location】On the radial side of the index finger, about 0.1 cun posterior to the corner of the nail (Fig. 19).

【Indications】Toothache, sore throat, swelling of the submandibular region, numbness of fingers, febrile diseases, loss of consciousness.

【Method】Puncture obliquely 0.1 inch, or prick with three-edged needle to cause bleeding.

商　陽　（しょうよう）

【部位】示指の橈側、爪甲角より後方約0.1寸（図19）。

【主治】歯痛、咽喉腫痛、顎腫、指のしびれ、熱性病、昏厥（一時性昏暈と昏迷の二つの症状を含む）。

【刺灸法】0.1寸斜刺し、あるいは三稜針で瀉血する。

合　谷

【位置】在第1、2掌骨之间，约当第2掌骨桡侧之中点。或以一手拇指的指关节横纹正对另一手的拇食指之间的指蹼缘上，当拇指尖所指处是穴（图20）。

【主治】头痛，目赤肿痛，鼻衄，齿痛，面肿，咽喉肿痛，指挛，臂痛，口眼歪斜，热病无汗，多汗，闭经，滞产，痢疾。

【刺灸法】直刺0.5～0.8寸；可灸。

Hegu

【Location】Between the 1st and 2nd metacarpal bones, approximately in the middle of the 2nd metacarpal

— 47 —

bone on the radial side. Or place in coincident position the transverse crease of the interphalangeal joint of the thumb with the margin of the web between the thumb and the index finger of the other hand. The point is where the tip of the thumb touches (Fig. 20).

【Indications】 Headache, redness with swelling and pain of the eye, epistaxis, toothache, facial swelling, sore throat, contracture of fingers, pain of the arm, trismus, facial paralysis, febrile diseases with anhidrosis, hidrosis, amenorrhea, delayed labour, dysentery.

【Method】 Puncture perpendicularly 0.5～0.8 inch. Moxibustion is applicable.

合 谷 （ごうこく）

【部位】第1、2中手骨の間、第2中手骨中央橈側にとる。または拇指の指関節横紋をもう一方手の拇指と示指の付根にあわせ、拇指先の指すところ（図20）。

【主治】頭痛、目の腫脹痛、鼻血、歯痛、顔面腫、咽喉腫脹痛、指の痙攣、上肢痛、口と目の歪み、熱性病、無汗、多汗、無月経、難産、赤痢。

【刺灸法】0.5～0.8寸直刺し、灸ができる。

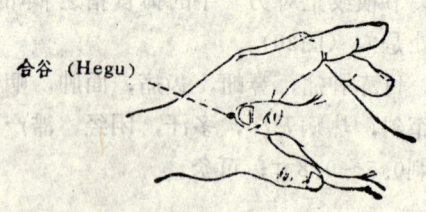

図(Fig.)20

曲　池

　　【位置】屈肘，肘横纹外端凹陷处，当尺泽与肱骨外上髁连线之中点（图21）。
　　【主治】肘臂痛，上肢不遂，瘰疬，风疹，腹痛，吐泻，痢疾，热病，咽喉肿痛。
　　【刺灸法】直刺1～1.5寸；可灸。

Quchi

【Location】When the elbow is flexed, the point is in the depression at the lateral end of the transverse cubital crease, midpoint between Chize and the lateral epicondyle of the humerus(Fig.21).

【Indications】Pain of the elbow and arm, motor impairment of the upper extremities, scrofula, urticaria, abdominal pain, vomiting, diarrhea, dysentery, febrile disease, sore throat.

【Method】Puncture perpendicularly 1.0～1.5 inches. Moxibustion is applicable.

　　曲　池　（きょくち）

　　【部位】肘を曲げて、肘横紋外端の陥凹にあり、尺沢と上腕骨外側上髁の連結線の中点にあたる（図21）。
　　【主治】肘腕の痛み、上肢麻痺、瘰癧、みっかばしか、腹痛、吐瀉、赤痢、熱性病、咽喉腫痛。
　　【刺灸法】1～1.5寸直刺し、灸ができる。

肩　髃

【位置】肩峰前下方，三角肌上部的中央。当上臂外展至水平位时，出现二个凹陷，在前方的凹陷是本穴（图21）。
【主治】肩臂痛，上肢不遂，风疹，瘰疬。
【刺灸法】向下斜刺0.6～1.2寸；可灸。
Jianyu
【Location】Anteroinferior to the acromion, in the middle of the upper portion of m. deltoideus. When the arm is in full abduction, the point is in the anterior depression of the two depressions appearing at the anterior border of the acromioclavicular joint (Fig.21).
【Indications】Pain of the shoulder and arm, motor impairment of the upper extremities, rubella, scrofula.
【Method】Puncture obliquely downward 0.6～1.2 inches. Moxibustion is applicable.

肩　髃　（けんぐう）

【部位】肩峰前下方、三角筋上部の中央にとる。上腕を水平位に外転するとき現れる二つの陥凹の前方の陥凹部（図21）。
【主治】肩腕痛，上肢麻痺，みっかばしか，瘰癧。
【刺灸法】0.6～1.2寸下に向けて斜刺し，灸ができる。

迎　香

【位置】在与鼻翼外缘中点平齐的鼻唇沟里取之（图19）。
【主治】鼻塞，鼻衄，鼻渊，口角歪斜，面痒，面肿。

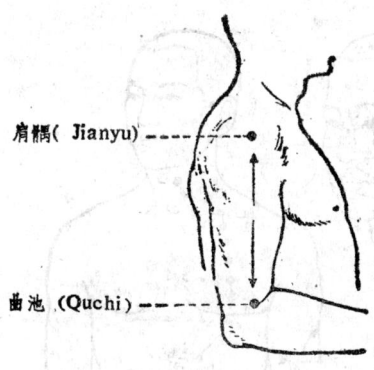

图(Fig.)21

【刺灸法】向下或斜刺0.3寸。

Yingxiang

【Location】In the nasolabial groove, at the level of the midpoint of the lateral border of ala nasi (Fig.19).

【Indications】Nasal obstruction, epistaxis, rhinorrhea, deviation of the mouth, itching and swelling of the face.

【Method】Puncture obliquely downward 0.3 inch.

迎 香 （げいこう）

【部位】鼻翼外縁中点と同じ水平線にある、鼻唇溝に取る（図19）。

【主治】鼻つまり、鼻血、口角の歪み、顔面搔痒感、顔面腫。

【刺灸法】0.3寸下に向け，あるいは斜刺する。

3. 足阳明胃经　经脉循行（图22）。
The Stomach Channel of Foot-Yangming

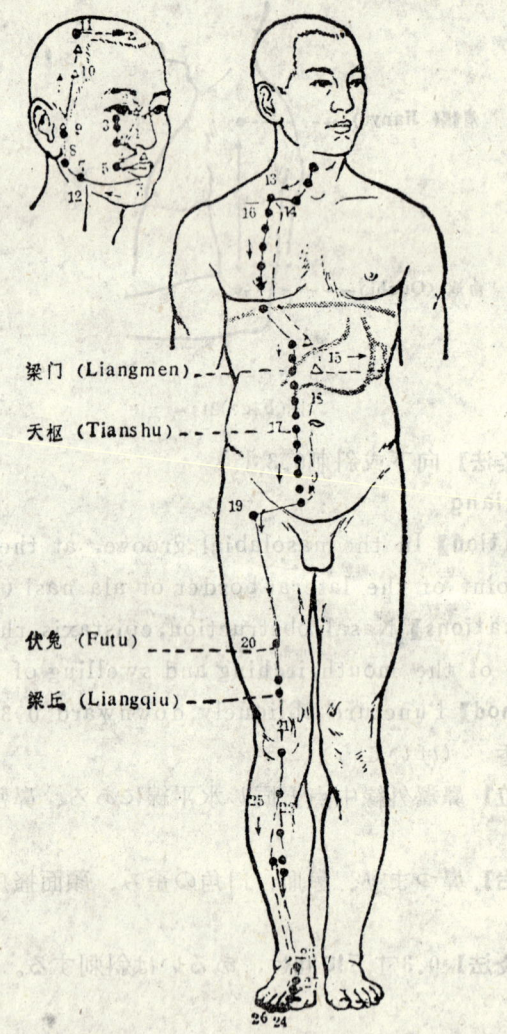

图(Fig.)22 足阳明胃经循行示意图
(The Stomach Channe of Foot-Yangming)

Channel Course (Fig.22).

足の陽明胃経　その経脈の循行は（図22）のようである。

地　仓

【位置】在口角外侧，巨髎穴的直下方（图23）。
【主治】口角歪斜，流涎，眼睑瞤动。
【刺灸法】针尖斜向颊车，针0.5～1寸；可灸。

Dicang

【Location】Lateral to the corner of the mouth, directly below Nose-Juliao(Fig.23).

【Indications】Deviation of the mouth, salivation, twitching of eyelids.

【Method】Puncture obliquely 0.5～1.0 inch with the tip of the needle directed towards Jiache. Moxibustion is applicable.

地　倉（ちそう）

【部位】口角の外側、巨髎の直下方にある（図23）。
【主治】口角の歪み、流涎、顔面神経痙攣。
【刺灸法】頰車に向けて0.5～1寸刺す、灸ができる。

颊　车

【位置】在下颌角的前上方一横指，咬肌附着部，上下齿咬紧时出现肌肉隆起（图23）。
【主治】口眼歪斜，颊肿，齿痛，牙关紧闭，颈项强痛，痄

— 53 —

腮。

【刺灸法】直刺0.3～0.5寸，或向地仓斜刺；可灸。

Jiache

【Location】One finger-breadth anterior and superior to the lower angle of the mandible where m.masseter attaches at the prominence of the muscle when the teeth are clenched (Fig.23).

【Indications】Facial paralysis, swelling of the cheek, toothache, trismus, pain and stiffness of the neck, mumps.

【Method】Puncture perpendicularly 0.3～0.5 inch or obliquely towards Dicang. Moxibustion is applicable.

頰車　（きょうしゃ）

【部位】下顎角の前上方一横指、咬筋愈着部、歯をくいしばる時に現れる筋肉隆起処にある（図23）。

【主治】口と目の歪み、頬腫、歯痛、牙関緊閉、頸項強痛、耳下腺炎。

【刺灸法】直刺0.3～0.5寸、或は地倉に向けて斜刺し、灸ができる。

下　关

【位置】颧弓下缘，下颌骨髁状突之前方，呈现凹陷处，闭口取穴（图23）。

【主治】耳聋，耳鸣，聤耳，口眼歪斜，齿痛，牙关开合不利。

【刺灸法】直刺0.3～0.5寸；可灸。

Xiaguan

【Location】In the depression at the lower border of the zygomatic arch, anterior to the condyloid process of the mandible. This point is located with the mouth closed (Fig. 23).

【Indications】Deafness, tinnitus, otorrhea, facial paralysis, toothache, motor impairment of the jaw.

【Method】Puncture perpendicularly 0.3～0.5 inch. Moxibustion is applicable.

下関　（げかん）

【部位】頬骨弓下縁、下顎関節突起の前方陥凹部、口を閉じて取る（図23）。

【主治】難聴、耳鳴、耳垢が原因の難聴、口と目の歪み、歯痛、口のあけしめがきかない。

【刺灸法】0.3～0.5寸直刺し、灸ができる。

头　维

【位置】在额角发际上5分；督脉旁开4.5寸（图23）。

【主治】头痛，目眩，目痛，迎风流泪。

【刺灸法】针尖向下或向后，沿皮刺0.5～1寸。

Touwei

【Location】0.5 cun within the anterior hairline at the corner of the forehead, 4.5 cun lateral to the Du Channel (Fig. 23).

【Indications】Headache, blurring of vision, ophthalmalgia, lacrimation when attacked by wind.

【Method】Puncture 0.5～1.0 inch along the scalp with the tip of the needle directed horizontally upward or downward.

頭維 (ずい)

【部位】前頭角の髪際の上0.5寸、督脈より横4.5寸のところにある（図23）。

【主治】頭痛、目眩、目痛、流涙。

【刺灸法】針先を下、あるいは後に向け、皮膚に沿って0.5～1寸刺す。

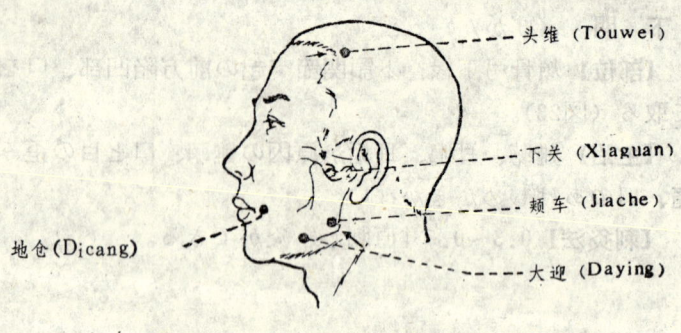

図(Fig.)23

梁門

【位置】在脐上4寸，中脘穴旁开2寸（图22）。

【主治】胃痛，呕吐，食欲不振，大便溏。

【刺灸法】直刺0.7～1寸；可灸。

Liangmen

【Location】4 cun above the umbilicus, 2 cun lateral to Zhongwan(Fig.22).

【Indications】Gastric pain, vomiting, anorexia, loose stools.

【Method】Puncture perpendicularly 0.7〜1.0 inch. Moxibustion is applicable.

梁　門　（りょうもん）

【部位】臍の上4寸、中脘の外側2寸にある（図22）。

【主治】嘔吐、胃痛、食欲不振、軟便。

【刺灸法】0.7〜1寸直刺し、灸ができる。

天　枢

【位置】脐中旁开2寸（图22）。

【主治】腹痛，泄泻，痢疾，便秘，肠鸣，腹胀，水肿，月经不调。

【刺灸法】直刺0.7〜1.2寸；可灸。

Tianshu

【Location】2 cun lateral to the centre of the umbilicus (Fig. 22).

【Indications】Abdominal pain, diarrhea, dysentery, constipation, borborygmus, abdominal distension, edema, irregular menstruation.

【Method】Puncture perpendicularly 0.7〜1.2 inches. Moxibustion is applicable.

天　枢　（てんすう）

【部位】臍の外側2寸にある（図22）。

【主治】腹痛、下痢、赤痢、便秘、腸鳴、腹膨満感、水腫、月経不順。

【刺灸法】0.7〜1.2寸直刺し、灸ができる。

伏 兔

【位置】在髌骨外上缘上6寸，髂前上棘与髌骨外缘的连线上（图22）。

【主治】腰胯痛，膝冷，下肢麻痹，脚气。

【刺灸法】直刺1～1.5寸；可灸。

Futu

【Location】6 cun above the laterosuperior border of the patella, on the line connecting the anterior superior iliac spine and lateral border of the patella (Fig. 22).

【Indications】Pain in the lumbar and iliac region, coldness of the knee, paralysis or motor impairment and pain of the lower extremities, beriberi.

【Method】Puncture perpendicularly 1.0～1.5 inches. Moxibustion is applicable.

伏 兎 （ふくと）

【部位】膝蓋骨外上縁の上6寸、腸骨前上棘と膝蓋骨外縁の連結線上にある（図22）。

【主治】腰痛、膝冷感、下肢麻痺、脚気。

【刺灸法】1～1.5寸直刺し、灸ができる。

梁 丘

【位置】髌骨外上缘上2寸（图22）。

【主治】膝肿痛，下肢不遂，胃痛，乳痈。

【刺灸法】直刺0.5～1寸；可灸。

Liangqiu

【Location】 2 cun above the laterosuperior border of the patella(Fig.22).

【Indications】 Pain and swelling of the knee, motor impairment of the lower extremities, gastric pain, mastitis.

【Method】 Puncture perpendicularly 0.5～1.0 inch. Moxibustion is applicable.

梁　丘　(りょうきゅう)
【部位】膝蓋骨外上縁の上2寸にある（図22）。
【主治】膝腫痛、下肢麻痺、胃痛、乳腺炎。
【刺灸法】0.5～1寸直刺し、灸ができる。

犊　鼻（又名外膝眼）

【位置】屈膝，当髌骨下髌韧带外侧凹陷中（图24）。
【主治】膝痛，麻木，屈伸不利，脚气。
【刺灸法】针尖略向内侧斜刺0.7～1寸；可灸。

Dubi (Also Known as External Xiyan)

【Location】 Ask the patient to flex the knee. The point is in the depression below the patella and lateral to the patellar ligament(Fig.24).

【Indications】 Pain, numbness and motor impairment of the knee, beriberi.

【Method】 Puncture obliquely 0.7～1.0 inch with the needle directed slightly towards the medial side. Moxibustion is applicable.

犊　鼻　(とくび)（外膝眼ともいう）

【部位】膝を曲げて、膝蓋骨下膝蓋靱帯外側の陥凹にある（図24）。

【主治】膝の痛み、しびれ、屈伸不便、脚気。

【刺灸法】針先を内側に少し向けて0.7～1寸斜刺し、灸ができる。

足三里

【位置】在犊鼻下3寸，距脛骨前嵴一横指（图24）。

【主治】胃痛，呕吐，腹胀，完谷不化，肠鸣，泄泻，便秘，痢疾，乳痈，头晕，癫狂，半身不遂，脚气，膝脛酸痛。

【刺灸法】直刺0.5～1.3寸；可灸。

Zusanli

【Location】3 cun below Dubi, one finger-breadth from the anterior crest of the tibia (Fig. 24).

【Indications】Gastric pain, vomiting, abdominal distension, indigestion, borborygmus, diarrhea, constipation, dysentery, mastitis, dizziness, mental disorders, hemiplegia, beriberi, aching of the knee joint and leg.

【Method】Puncture perpendicularly 0.5～1.3 inches. Moxibustion is applicable.

足三里　（あしさんり）

【部位】犊鼻の下3寸、脛骨前縁から一横指のところにある（図24）。

【主治】胃痛、嘔吐、腹脹、消化不良、腸鳴、下痢、便秘、赤痢、乳腺炎、眩暈、癲癇、半身麻痺、脚気、膝と小腿の疼痛。

【刺灸法】0.5～1.3寸直刺し、灸ができる。

丰　隆

　　【位置】外踝前上8寸，在条口穴的后方约一横指（图24）。
　　【主治】胸痛，气喘，痰多，咽喉肿痛，下肢痿痹、肿痛，头痛，头晕，癫狂，痫证。
　　【刺灸法】直刺0.5～1寸；可灸。

Fenglong

〖Location〗 8 cun superior and anterior to the external malleolus, about one finger-breadth posterior to Tiaokou(Fig.24).

〖Indications〗 Chest pain, asthma, excessive sputum, sore throat, muscular atrophy, motor impairment, pain, paralysis or swelling of the lower extremities, headache, dizziness, mental disorders, epilepsy.

〖Method〗 Puncture perpendicularly 0.5～1.0 inch. Moxibustion is applicable.

　　豊　隆　（ほうりゅう）
　　【部位】外踝前上8寸、条口の後方約一横指のところにある（図24）。
　　【主治】胸痛、喘息、痰が多い、咽喉腫痛、下肢麻痺、腫痛、頭痛、眩暈、癲狂、ひきつけ。
　　【刺灸法】0.5～1寸直刺し、灸ができる。

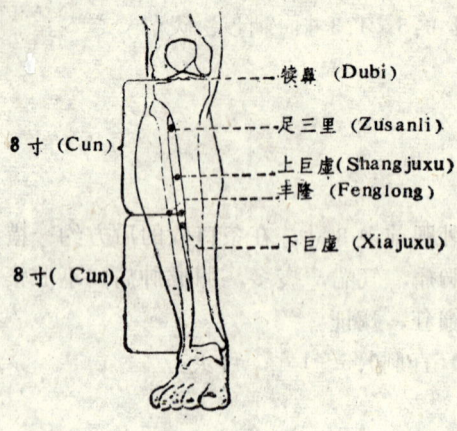

图(Fig.)24

解 溪

【位置】在足背与小腿交界处，当趾长伸肌腱与踇长伸肌腱之间，约与外踝高点相平（图25）。

【主治】头面浮肿，头痛，眩晕，腹胀，便秘，下肢痿痹，癫证。

【刺灸法】直刺0.5～0.7寸；可灸。

Jiexi

【Location】At the junction of the dorsum of foot and the leg, between the tendons of m. extensor digitorum longus and hallucis longus, approximately at the level of the tip of the external malleolus(Fig.25).

【Indications】Edema of the head and face, headache, dizziness and vertigo, abdominal distension, constipation, muscular atrophy, motor impairment, pain and paralysis of the lower extremities, mental disorder of depressive type.

【Method】Puncture perpendicularly 0.5～0.7 inch. Moxibustion is applicable.

解　谿　　（かいけい）

【部位】足背と小腿の交界、長指伸筋腱と長蹈指伸筋腱の間にあたる。外踝尖端との水平線上にある（図25）。

【主治】顔面浮腫、頭痛、眩暈、腹脹、便秘、下肢麻痺、癲症。

【刺灸法】0.5～0.7寸直刺し、灸ができる。

内　庭

【位置】在足背第2、3趾的趾縫間，当第2趾跖关节前外方凹陷中（图25）。

【主治】齿痛，口角歪斜，鼻衄，腹痛，腹胀，泄泻，痢疾，足背肿痛，热病。

【刺灸法】直刺0.3～0.5寸；可灸。

Neiting

【Location】Proximal to the web margin between the 2nd and 3rd toes, in the depression distal and lateral to the 2nd metatarsodigital joint (Fig.25).

【Indication】Toothache, deviation of the mouth, epistaxis, abdominal pain or distension, diarrhea, dysentery, pain and swelling of the dorsum of foot, febrile diseases.

【Method】Puncture perpendicularly 0.3～0.5 inch. Moxibustion is applicable.

内　庭　（ないてい）

【部位】足背第2、3指の結合部にあり、第2中足趾関節前外方陥凹にあたる（図25）。

【主治】歯痛、口角の歪み、鼻血、腹痛、腹膨満、下痢、赤痢、足背腫痛、熱性病。

【刺灸法】0.3～0.5寸直刺し、灸ができる。

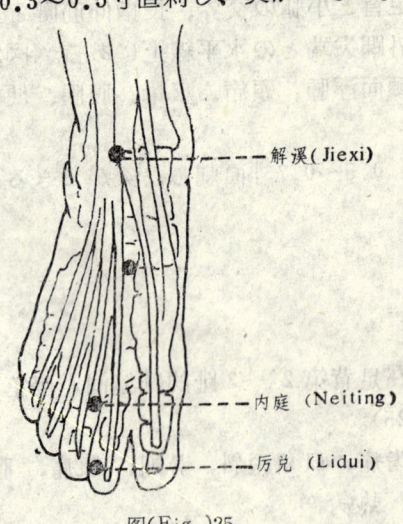

図(Fig.)25

厉　兑

【位置】在第2趾外側，趾甲角后1分许（图25）。

【主治】面肿，口角歪斜，齿痛，鼻衄，胸腹胀满，足胫寒冷，热病，多梦，癫狂。

【刺灸法】斜刺0.1寸；可灸。

Lidui

【Location】On the lateral side of the 2nd toe, about

0.1 cun posterior to the corner of nail (Fig.25).

【Indications】 Facial swelling, deviation of the mouth, toothache, epistaxis, distending sensation of the chest and abdomen, cold in the leg and foot, febrile diseases, dream-disturbed sleep, mental confusion.

【Method】 Puncture obliquely 0.1 inch. Moxibustion is applicable.

歷兌　（れいだ）

【部位】第2趾骨の外側、爪甲角の後約0.1寸のところにある（図25）。

【主治】顔面浮腫、口角の歪み、歯痛、鼻血、胸腹膨満、足腿冷感、熱性病、多夢、癲狂。

【刺灸法】0.1寸斜刺し、灸ができる。

4. 足太阴脾经　经脉循行（图26）。
The Spleen Channel of Foot-Taiyin Channel Course (Fig.26).

足の太陰脾経　その経脈の循行は（図26）のようである。

隐　白

【位置】足踇趾内側，趾甲角后1分许（图27）。
【主治】腹胀，崩漏，癫狂，多梦，惊风。
【刺灸法】斜刺0.1寸；可灸。
Yinbai
【Location】 On the medial side of the big toe, about 0.1 cun posterior to the corner of the nail (Fig.27).

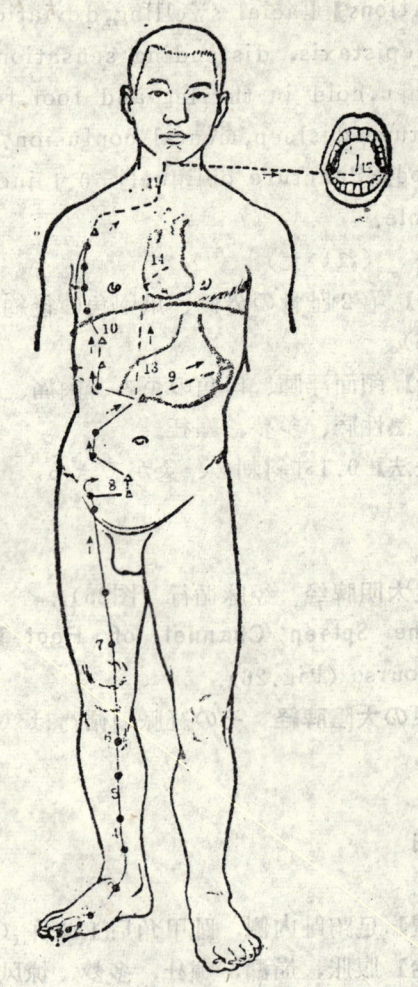

图(Fig.)26 足太阴脾经循行示意图
(The Spleen Channel of Foot-Taiyin)

— 66 —

【Indication】 Abdominal distension, uterine bleeding, mental disorders, dream-disturbed sleep, convulsion.

【Method】 Puncture obliquely 0.1 inch. Moxibustion is applicable.

隠白 （いんぱく）

【部位】足蹈趾の内側、爪甲角の後約0.1寸のところにある（図27）。

【主治】腹脹、崩漏、癲狂、多夢、ひきつけ。

【刺灸法】0.1寸斜刺し、灸ができる。

三阴交

【位置】内踝高点直上3寸，胫骨后缘当内踝与阴陵泉的连线上（图27）。

【主治】肠鸣，腹胀，大便溏泄，完谷不化，月经不调，崩漏，带下，阴挺，闭经，不孕，难产，遗精，阴部痛，疝气，小便不利，遗尿，下肢痿痹，失眠。

【刺灸法】直刺0.5～1寸；可灸。

Sanyinjiao

【Location】 3 cun directly above the tip of the medial malleolus, on the posterior border of the tibia, on the line drawn from the medial malleolus to Yinlingquan (Fig. 27).

【Indications】 Borborygmus, abdominal distension, loose stools with undigested food, irregular menstruation, uterine bleeding, leukorrhea, prolapse of uterus, amenorrhea, sterility, difficult labour, seminal emission, pain of the external genitalia, hernia, dysuria, enuresis, muscular atrophy,motor impairment and paralysis and pain of the lower extremities,insomnia.

【Method】Puncture perpendicularly 0.5～1.0 inch. Moxibustion is applicable.

三陰交 （さんいんこう）

【部位】内踝隆起の上3寸、脛骨後縁、内踝と陰陵泉の連結線上にあたる（図27）。

【主治】腸鳴、腹脹、軟便、消化不良、月経不順、月経過多、白帯下、子宮脱垂、無月経、不妊症、難産、遺精、陰部痛、脱腸、小便不暢、遺尿、下肢麻痺、不眠症。

【刺灸法】0.5～1寸直刺し、灸ができる。

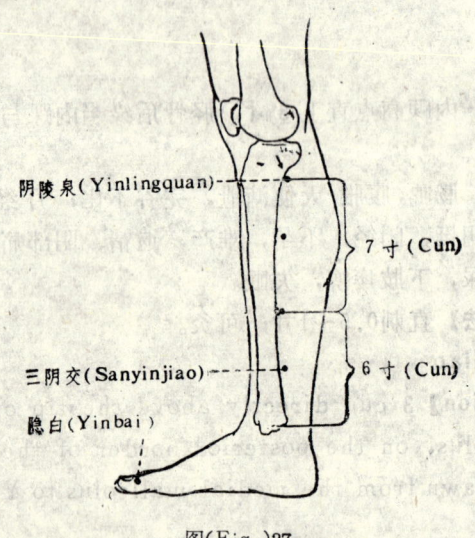

图(Fig.)27

阴陵泉

【位置】在胫骨内髁下缘，胫骨后缘和腓肠肌之间凹陷处

（图27）。

【主治】腹胀，水肿，黄疸，泄泻，小便不利或失禁，阴部痛，遗精，膝痛。

【刺灸法】直刺0.5～1寸；可灸。

Yinlingquan

【Location】 On the lower border of the medial condyle of the tibia, in the depression between the posterior border of the tibia and m.gastrocnemius (Fig.27).

【Indications】 Abdominal distension, edema, jaundice, diarrhea, dysuria, incontinence of urine, pain of the external genitalia, seminal emission, pain in the knee.

【Method】 Puncture perpendicularly 0.5～1.0 inch. Moxibustion is applicable.

陰陵泉　（いんりょうせん）

【部位】脛骨内側踝下縁、脛骨後縁と腓腹筋の間の陷凹にある（図27）。

【主治】腹脹、水腫、黄疸、下痢、排尿困難及び尿失禁、外生殖器疼痛、遺精、膝痛。

【刺灸法】0.5～1寸直刺し、灸ができる。

血 海

【位置】屈膝，髌骨内上缘上2寸，当股四头肌内侧头的隆起处，或以手掌按其膝盖，二至五指向膝上，拇指偏向膝内侧，当大指尖端所指处是穴（图28）。

【主治】月经不调，痛经，闭经，崩漏，股内侧痛，皮肤湿疹，风疹。

【刺灸法】直刺0.7～1.2寸；可灸。

Xuehai

【Location】When knee is flexed, the point is 2 cun above the mediosuperior border of the patella, on the bulge of the medial portion of m. quadriceps femoris. Another way to locate this point is to cup your right palm to the patient's left knee, with the thumb on its medial side and the other four fingers directed proximally. The point is where the tip of your thumb rests (Fig. 28).

【Indications】Irregular menstruation, dysmenorrhea, amenorrhea, uterine bleeding, pain in the medial aspect of the thigh, eczema, urticaria.

【Method】Puncture perpendicularly 0.7～1.2 inches. Moxibustion is applicable.

血海 （けっかい）

【部位】膝を曲げて、膝蓋骨内上縁の上2寸、大腿四頭筋内側頭の隆起処にあたる。あるいは掌をその膝蓋にあて、人差指から小指までは膝の上に、拇指は膝内側に向け、拇指先のあたるところにある（図28）。

【主治】月経不順、生理痛、無月経、月経過多、大腿内側痛、皮膚湿疹、みっかばしか。

【刺灸法】0.7～1.2寸直刺し、灸ができる。

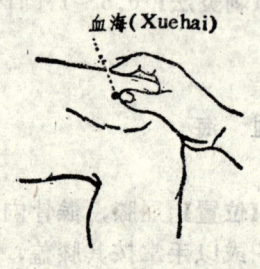

図(Fig.)28

5. 手少阴心经　经脉循行（図29）。
　　The Heart Channel of Hand-Shaoyin

Channel Course (Fig. 29).

手の少陰心経 その経脈の循行は（図29）のようである。

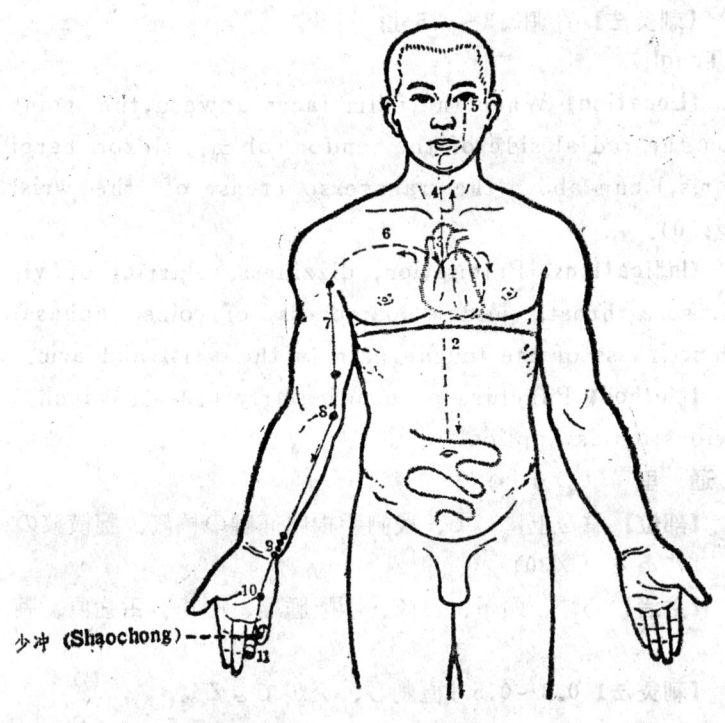

少冲 (Shaochong)

図(Fig.)29 手少阴心经循行示意图
(The Heart Channel of Hand-Shaoyin)

通 里

【位置】仰掌，在尺侧腕屈肌腱之桡侧，腕横纹上1寸

（图30）。

【主治】心悸怔忡，头晕，目眩，咽喉肿痛，暴瘖，舌强不语，腕臂痛。

【刺灸法】直刺0.3～0.5寸；可灸。

Tongli

【Location】When the palm faces upward, the point is on the radial side of the tendon of m. flexor carpi ulnaris, 1 cun above the transverse crease of the wrist (Fig. 30).

【Indications】Palpitation, dizziness, blurring of vision, sore throat, sudden hoarseness of voice, aphasai with stiffness of the tongue, pain in the wrist and arm.

【Method】Puncture perpendicularly 0.3～0.5 inch. Moxibustion is applicable.

通里 （つうり）

【部位】掌を上にして、尺側手根屈筋腱の橈側、腕横紋の上1寸にある（図30）。

【主治】心悸、頭暈、目眩、咽喉腫痛、嗄声、舌強直、腕痛。

【刺灸法】0.3～0.5寸直刺し、灸ができる。

神 门

【位置】在豌豆骨与尺骨关节部的腕横纹上，当尺侧腕屈肌腱之桡侧凹陷中（图30）。

【主治】心痛，心烦，癫狂，痫证，健忘，怔忡，惊悸，失眠，目黄，胁痛，掌中热。

【刺灸法】直刺0.3～0.5寸；可灸。

Shenmen

【Location】 On the transverse crease of the wrist, in the articular region between the pisiform bone and the ulna, in the depression on the radial side of the tendon of m. flexor carpi ulnaris (Fig. 30).

【Indications】 Cardiac pain, irritability, mental disorders, epilepsy, poor memory, palpitation, panic, insomnia, yellowish sclera, pain in the hypochondriac region, feverish sensation in the palm.

【Method】 Puncture perpendicularly 0.3～0.5 inch. Moxibustion is applicable.

神門 （しんもん）

【部位】豆状骨と尺骨関節部の腕横紋にあり、尺側手根屈筋腱の橈側陥凹にあたる（図30）。

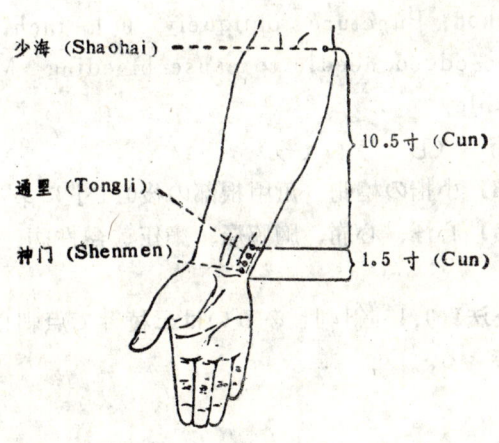

図(Fig.)30

【主治】心痛、心煩、癲狂、ひきつけ、健忘、怔忡（心臓のはげしく拍動する症状）、驚悸、不眠症、目黄、脇痛、掌中熱。

— 73 —

【刺灸法】0.3～0.5寸直刺し、灸ができる。

少　冲

【位置】小指桡侧，指甲角后1分许（图29）。
【主治】心悸，心痛，胸胁痛，癫狂，热病，昏厥。
【刺灸法】斜刺0.1寸或三棱针点刺出血；可灸。

Shaochong

[Location] On the radial side of the little finger, about 0.1 cun posterior to the corner of the nail (Fig. 29).

[Indications] Palpitation, cardiac pain, pain in the chest and hypochondriac region, mental disorders, febrile diseases, loss of consciousness.

[Method] Puncture obliquely 0.1 inch, or prick with three-edged needle to cause bleeding. Moxibustion is applicable.

少　衝　（しょうしょう）
【位部】小指の橈側、爪甲根部の後0.1寸にある（図29）。
【主治】心悸、心痛、胸脇痛、癲狂、熱性病、昏睡或は一時性昏暈。
【刺灸法】0.1寸斜刺しあるいは三稜針で点刺して瀉血する。灸ができる。

6. 手太阳小肠经　经脉循行（图31）。
The Small Intestine Channel of Hand-Taiyang
Channel Course (Fig. 31).

手の太陽小腸経 その経脈の循行は（図31）のようである。

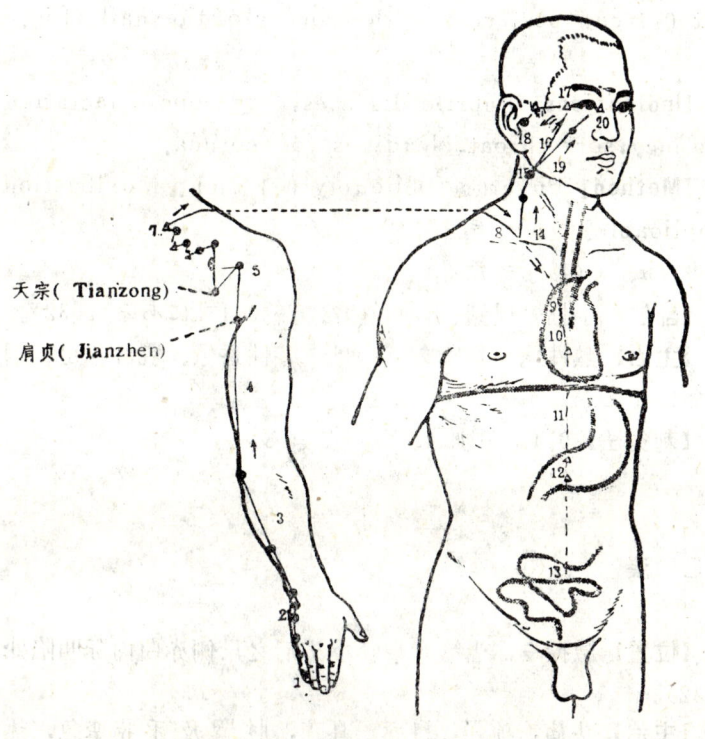

図(Fig.)31 手太阳小肠经循行示意图
(The Small Intestine Channel of Hand-Taiyang)

少 泽

【位置】在小指尺側，爪甲角后1分许（图32）。
【主治】热病，昏厥，乳汁少，咽喉肿痛，目翳。

【刺灸法】斜刺0.1寸；可灸。

Shaoze

[Location] On the ulnar side of the little finger, about 0.1 cun posterior to the corner of the nail (Fig. 32).

[Indications] Febrile diseases, syncope lactation deficiency, sore throat, cloudiness of cornea.

[Method] Puncture obliquely 0.1 inch. Moxibustion is applicable.

少沢　（しょうたく）

【部位】小指の尺側、爪甲角の後方約0.1寸にある（図32）。

【主治】熱性病、昏睡あるいは一時性昏暈、乳汁不足、咽喉腫痛、そこひ。

【刺灸法】0.1寸斜刺し、灸ができる。

后　溪

【位置】微握拳，当第5掌骨小头后之尺侧赤白肉际凹陷处（图32）。

【主治】头痛，项强，目赤，耳聋，肘臂及手指挛急，热病，癫痫，疟疾，盗汗。

【刺灸法】直刺0.5～0.7寸；可灸。

Houxi

[Location] When a loose fist is made, the point is proximal to the head of the 5th metacarpal bone on the ulnar side, in the depression at the junction of the red and white skin (Fig. 32).

[Indications] Headache, neck rigidity, congestion of

the eye,deafness, contracture and twitching of the elbow,arm and fingers,febrile diseases, epilepsy,malaria, night sweating.

【Method】Puncture perpendicularly 0.5~0.7 inch. Moxibustion is applicable.

後　谿（こうけい）

【部位】やや拳を握って、第5中手骨頭の後尺側、赤白皮膚色の肌目の陥凹にあたる（図32）。

【主治】頭痛、項強直、赤目、難聴、肘腕及び指の痙攣、熱性病、癲癇、マラリヤ、寝汗。

【刺灸法】0.5~0.7寸直刺し、灸ができる。

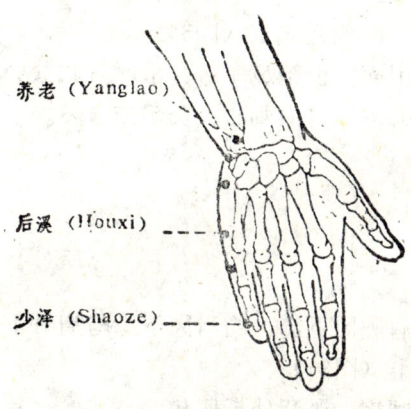

図(Fig.)32

肩　贞

【位置】在肩关节后下方，上臂内收时，从腋纹头上1寸处取穴（图31）。

— 77 —

【主治】肩胛痛，手臂痛不举。
【刺灸法】直刺0.5～1寸；可灸。
　Jianzhen

　【Location】 Posterior and inferior to the shoulder joint. When the arm is adducted, the point is 1 cun above the posterior end of the axillary fold (Fig.31).

　【Indications】 Pain in the scapular region, pain and motor impairment of the hand and arm.

　【Method】 Puncture perpendicularly 0.5～1.0 inch. Moxibustion is applicable.

　肩　貞　（けんてい）
　【部位】肩関節の後下方にあり、前腕を下げ脇につけ、腋窩横紋端の上1寸に取穴する（図31）。
　【主治】肩甲痛、上腕が痛く、挙げられない。
　【刺灸法】0.5～1寸直刺し、灸ができる。

　天　宗

　【位置】在肩胛冈下窝，约当冈下缘与肩胛下角间的上1/3与中1/3的交点上（图31）。
　【主治】肩胛痛，肘臂外后侧痛。
　【刺灸法】斜刺0.5～1寸；可灸。
　Tianzong

　【Location】 In the infrascapular fossa, at the junction of the upper and middle third of the distance between the lower border of the scapular spine and the inferior angle of the scapula (Fig.31).

　【Indications】 Pain in the scapular region, pain in

the lateroposterior aspect of the elbow and arm.

【Method】 Puncture obliquely 0.5〜1.0 inch. Moxibustion is applicable.

天宗　（てんそう）

【部位】肩甲棘下窩、棘下縁と肩甲下角の間の上1/3と2/3の交叉点に当る（図31）。

【主治】肩甲痛、肘腕外後側痛。

【刺灸法】0.5〜1寸斜刺し、灸ができる。

听宫

【位置】在耳屏与下颌关节之间，微张口时呈凹陷处（图33）。

【主治】耳聋，耳鸣，聤耳。

【刺灸法】直刺0.3〜1寸；可灸。

Tinggong

【Location】 Between the tragus and the mandibular joint, where a depression is formed when the mouth is slightly open(Fig.33).

【Indications】 Deafness, tinnitus, otorrhea.

【Method】 Puncture perpendicularly 0.3〜1.0 inch. Moxibustion is applicable.

聴宮　（ちょうきゅう）

【部位】耳珠と下顎関節の間にあり、やや口をあけると陥凹のあるところ（図33）。

【主治】難聴、耳鳴、みみだれ。

【刺灸法】0.3〜1寸直刺し、灸ができる。

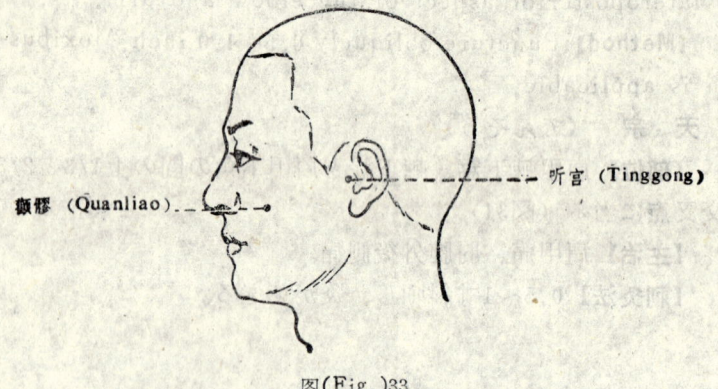

图(Fig.)33

7. 足太阳膀胱经 经脉循行（图34）。
The Urinary Bladder Channel of Foot-Taiyang Channel Course (Fig.34).
足の太陽膀胱経 その経脈の循行は（図34）のようである。

睛 明

【位置】闭目，在目内眦角上方0.1寸处（图35）。
【主治】目赤肿痛，见风流泪，眦痒，夜盲，色盲。
【刺灸法】沿眼眶边缘直刺0.3寸，不做大幅度的捻转和提插。

Jingming

[Location] 0.1 cun superior to the inner canthus. Ask the patient to close the eyes when locating the point (Fig.35).

[Indications] Redness, swelling and pain of the eye,

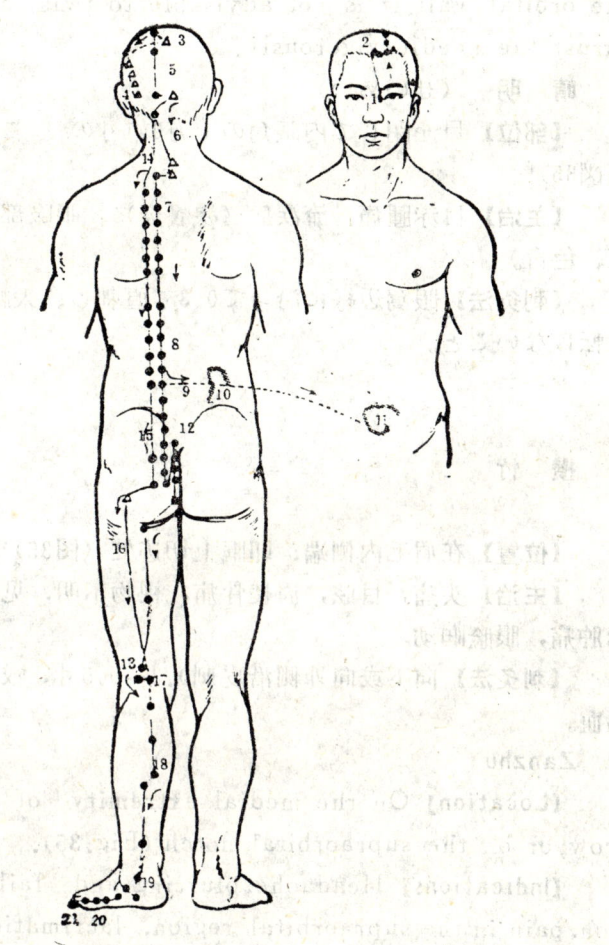

图(Fig.)34 足太阳膀胱经循行示意图
(The Urinary Bladder Channel of Foot-Taiyang)

lacrimation when attacked by wind, itching of the canthus, night blindness, colour blindness.

【Method】Puncture perpendicularly 0.3 inch along the orbital wall. It is not advisable to twist or lift and thrust the needle vigorously.

睛 明 （せいめい）

【部位】目を閉じて内眼角の上方0.1寸のところにある（図35）。

【主治】目赤腫痛、流涙症（涙嚢炎）、眼瞼部掻痒、夜盲症、色盲。

【刺灸法】眼窩辺縁に沿って0.3寸直刺し、大幅に提挿、捻転しないこと。

攢 竹

【位置】在眉毛内側端，即眶上切迹处（図35）。

【主治】头痛，目眩，眉棱骨痛，视物不明，见风流泪，目赤肿痛，眼睑瞤动。

【刺灸法】向下或向外側沿皮刺0.3～0.5寸，或三棱针点刺出血。

Zanzhu

【Location】On the medial extremity of the eyebrow, or on the supraorbital notch (Fig. 35).

【Indications】Headache, blurring and failing of vision, pain in the supraorbital region, lacrimation in face of wind, redness, swelling and pain of the eye, twitching of eyelids.

【Method】Puncture 0.3～0.5 inch horizontally along

the skin with the needle directed inferiorly or laterally, or prick with three-edged needle to cause bleeding.

攢竹 （さんちく）

【部位】眉毛内端、即ち眼窩上切痕のところにある（図35）。

【主治】頭痛、眩暈、視物不明、前額痛、流涙症、目赤腫痛、眼瞼痙攣。

【刺灸法】下に向ってあるいは外側に向け皮膚に沿って0.3～0.5寸刺す。または三稜針で点刺し、出血させる。

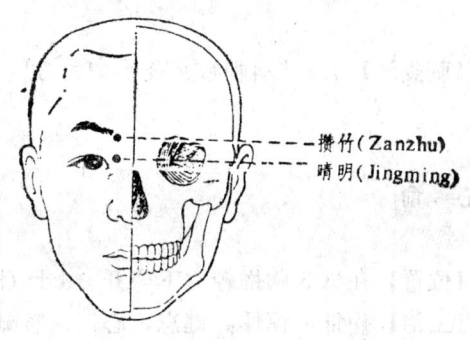

图(Fig.)35

肺 俞

【位置】在第3胸椎棘突下旁开1.5寸（图36）。

【主治】咳嗽，气喘，吐血，骨蒸潮热，盗汗。

【刺灸法】斜刺0.5寸；可灸。

Feishu

【Location】1.5 cun lateral to the lower border of

the spinous process of the 3rd thoracic vertebra(Fig. 36).

【Indications】Cough, asthma, hemoptysis, afternoon fever, night sweating.

【Method】Puncture obliquely 0.5 inch. Moxibustion is applicable.

肺兪　（はいゆ）

【部位】第3胸椎棘突起の外側1.5寸のところにある（図36）。

【主治】咳嗽、喘息、吐血、骨蒸潮熱（全身的な虚熱）、寝汗。

【刺灸法】0.5寸斜刺し、灸ができる。

心　兪

【位置】在第5胸椎棘突下旁开1.5寸（图36）。

【主治】痫证，惊悸，健忘，心烦，咳嗽，吐血。

【刺灸法】斜刺0.5寸；可灸。

Xinshu

【Location】1.5 cun lateral to the lower border of the spinous process of the 5th thoracic vertebra (Fig. 36).

【Indications】Epilepsy, panic palpitation, forgetfulness, irritability, cough, hemoptysis.

【Method】Puncture obliquely 0.5 inch. Moxibustion is applicable.

心兪　（しんゆ）

【部位】第5胸椎棘突起の外側1.5寸のところにある（図

36)。

【主治】ひきつけ、驚悸、健忘、心煩（胸部がほてってむかむかする）、咳嗽、吐血。

【刺灸法】0.5寸斜刺し、灸ができる。

膈　俞

【位置】在第7胸椎棘突下旁开1.5寸（图36）。

【主治】呕吐，呃逆，饮食不下，气喘，咳嗽，吐血，潮热，盗汗。

【刺灸法】斜刺0.5寸；可灸。

Geshu

【Location】 1.5 cun lateral to the lower border of the spinous process of the 7th thoracic vertebra (Fig. 36).

【Indications】 Vomiting, hiccup, difficulty in swallowing, asthma, cough, hemoptysis, afternoon fever, night sweating.

【Method】 Puncture obliquely 0.5 inch. Moxibustion is applicable.

膈　俞　（かくゆ）

【部位】第7胸椎棘突起の外側1.5寸のところにある（図36）。

【主治】嘔吐、吃逆、食道狭窄、喘息、咳嗽、吐血、潮熱、寝汗。

【刺灸法】0.5寸斜刺し、灸ができる。

肝　俞

【位置】第9胸椎棘突下旁开1.5寸（图36）。

【主治】黄疸，胁痛，吐血，鼻衄，目赤，目眩，夜盲，脊背痛，癫狂，痫证。

【刺灸法】斜刺0.5寸；可灸。

Ganshu

[Location] 1.5 cun lateral to the lower border of the spinous process of the 9th thoracic vertebra (Fig. 36).

[Indications] Jaundice, pain in the hypochondriac region, hematemesis, epistaxis, redness of the eye, blurring of vision, night blindness, pain in the back, mental confusion, epilepsy.

[Method] Puncture obliquely 0.5 inch. Moxibustion is applicable.

肝　俞　（かんゆ）

【部位】第9胸椎棘突起の外側1.5寸のところにある（図36）。

【主治】黄疸、脇痛、吐血、鼻血、目赤、目眩、夜盲症、背脊痛、癲狂、ひきつけ。

【刺灸法】0.5寸斜刺し、灸ができる。

脾　俞

【位置】第11胸椎棘突下旁开1.5寸（图36）。

【主治】腹胀，黄疸，呕吐，泄泻，痢疾，完谷不化，水肿，背痛。

【刺灸法】斜刺0.5寸；可灸。

Pishu

【Location】1.5 cun lateral to the lower border of the spinous process of the 11th thoracic vertebra (Fig. 36).

【Indications】Abdominal distension, jaundice, vomiting, diarrhea, dysentery, indigestion, edema, pain in the back.

【Method】Puncture obliquely 0.5 inch. Moxibustion is applicable.

脾俞　（ひゆ）

【部位】第11胸椎棘突起の外側1.5寸のところにある（図36）。

【主治】腹脹、黄疸、嘔吐、下痢、赤痢、消化不良、浮腫、背痛。

【刺灸法】0.5寸斜刺し、灸ができる。

腎俞

【位置】第2腰椎棘突下旁开1.5寸（图36）。

【主治】遗精，阳痿，遗尿，月经不调，白带，腰膝酸软，目昏，耳鸣，耳聋，水肿。

【刺灸法】直刺1～1.5寸；可灸。

Shenshu.

【Location】1.5 cun lateral to the lower border of the spinous process of the 2nd lumbar vertebra (Fig. 36).

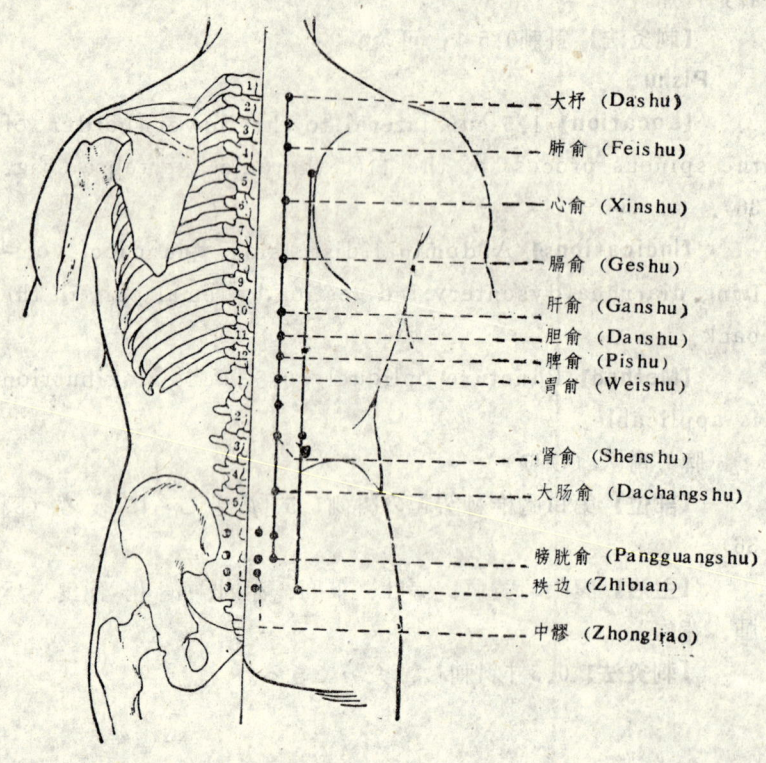

图(Fig.)36

【Indications】 Seminal emission, impotence, enuresis, irregular menstruation, leukorrhea, backache, weakness of the knee, blurring of vision, tinnitus, deafness, edema.

【Method】 Puncture perpendicularly 0.1～1.5 inches. Moxibustion is applicable.

腎　兪　（じんゆ）

【部位】第2腰椎棘突起の外側1.5寸のところにある（図

36)。

【主治】遺精、陰萎、遺尿、月経不順、帯下、腰膝がだるくて無力、のぼせ、耳鳴、難聴、水腫。

【刺灸法】1～1.5寸直刺し、灸ができる。

秩 边

【位置】胞盲直下方，督脉旁开3寸，约当骶管裂孔旁四横指处（图36）。

【主治】腰骶痛，痔疾，下肢痿痹。

【刺灸法】直刺1～1.5寸；可灸。

Zhibian

【Location】Directly below Baohuang, 3 cun lateral to Du channel, about 4 finger-breadths lateral to the hiatus of the sacrum (Fig.36).

【Indications】Pain in the lumbosacral region, hemorrhoids, muscular atrophy, motor impairment and pain of the lower extremities.

【Method】Puncture perpendicularly 1.0～1.5 inches. Moxibustion is applicable.

秩 辺 （ちっぺん）

【部位】胞盲穴の直下方、督脈の外側3寸の所。第4後仙骨孔より4横指のところにある（図36）。

【主治】腰仙部痛、痔症、下肢麻痺。

【刺灸法】1～1.5寸直刺し、灸ができる。

委 中

【位置】在腘窝横纹中央，当股二头肌腱与半腱肌肌腱之间，屈膝或俯卧取之（图37）。

【主治】腰痛，髋关节屈伸不利，腘筋挛急，下肢痿痹，半身不遂，腹痛，吐泻。

【刺灸法】直刺0.5～1.5寸，或三棱针点刺出血。

Weizhong

[Location] Midpoint of the transverse crease of the popliteal fossa, between the tendons of m. biceps femoris and m. semitendinosus. Locate the point in prone position or with flexed knee (Fig. 37).

[Indications] Low back pain, motor impairment of the hip joint, contracture of the tendons in the popliteal fossa, muscular atrophy, motor impairment and pain of the lower extremities, hemiplegia, abdominal pain, vomiting and diarrhea.

[Method] Puncture perpendicularly 0.5～1.5 inches, or prick with three-edged needle to cause bleeding.

委中　（いちゅう）

【部位】膝窩横紋の中点にあり、大腿二頭筋腱と半腱様筋腱との中間にあたる。膝を曲げ、あるいは伏臥位で取る（図37）。

【主治】腰痛、大腿関節屈伸障害、膝窩筋痙攣、下肢麻痺、半身不遂、腹痛、吐き下し（急性胃腸炎）。

【刺灸法】0.5～1.5寸直刺し、或は三稜針で点刺して出血させる。

承　山

【位置】在腓肠肌肌腹下，委中与跟腱的连线上，约当委中下8寸处（图37）。

【主治】腰痛，腿痛转筋，痔疾，便秘。
【刺灸法】直刺0.5～1寸；可灸。

Chengshan

【Location】Directly below the belly of m. gastrocnemius, on the line connecting Weizhong and tendo calcaneus, about 8 cun below Weizhong (Fig. 37).

【Indications】Low back pain, spasm of the gastrocnemius, hemorrhoids, constipation.

【Method】Puncture perpendicularly 0.5～1.0 inch. Moxibustion is applicable.

承 山 （しょうざん）

【部位】腓腹筋筋膜の下縁、委中穴とアキレス腱との連結線上にある。委中穴の下8寸のところにあたる（図37）。

【主治】腰痛、こむら返り（腓腹筋痙攣）、痔症、便秘。

【刺灸法】0.5～1寸直刺し、灸ができる。

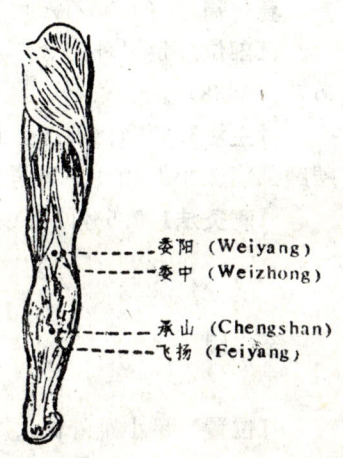

图(Fig.)37

昆 仑

【位置】在外踝与跟腱之中央凹陷部（图38）。

【主治】头痛，项强，目眩，鼻衄，肩臂拘急，腰痛，脚跟痛，小儿痫证，难产。

【刺灸法】直刺0.5寸；可灸。

Kunlun

【Location】In the depression between the external malleolus and tendo calcaneus (Fig. 38).

【Indications】Headache, neck rigidity, blurring of vision, epistaxis, spasm and pain of the shoulder and arm, backache, pain in the heel, epilepsy in children, difficult labour.

【Method】Puncture perpendicularly 0.5 inch. Moxibustion is applicable.

崑崙　（こんろん）

【部位】足外踝とアキレス腱との中点の陥凹したところにある（図38）。

【主治】頭痛、項部強直、目眩、鼻血、肩膊痙攣、腰痛、踝踵部痛、小児癇症、難産。

【刺灸法】0.5寸直刺し、灸ができる。

至　阴

【位置】足小趾外側，趾甲角后1分许（图38）。
【主治】头痛，鼻塞，鼻衄，目痛，足下热，难产。
【刺灸法】斜刺0.1寸；可灸。

Zhiyin

【Location】On the lateral side of the small toe, about 0.1 cun posterior to the corner of the nail (Fig. 38).

【Indications】Headache, nasal obstruction, epistaxis, ophthalmalgia, feverish sensation in sole, difficult labour.

【Method】Puncture obliquely 0.1 inch. Moxibustion is applicable.

至 陰　（しいん）

【部位】足の第5趾外側の爪甲角より後約0.1寸のところ（図38）。

【主治】頭痛、鼻つまり、鼻血、眼痛、足底熱感、難産。

【刺灸法】0.1寸斜刺し、灸ができる。

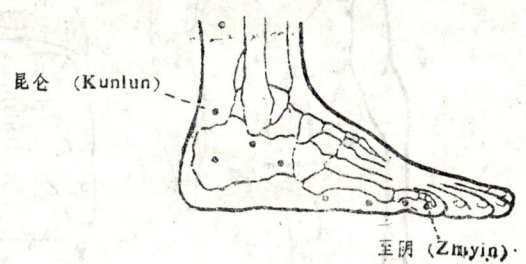

図(Fig.)38

8. 足少阴肾经　经脉循行（图39）。

The kidney Channel of Foot-Shaoyin Channel Course (Fig.39).

足の少陰腎経　その経脈の循行は（図39）のようである。

涌　泉

【位置】在足心，踡足时呈凹陷处，约当足底(去趾)前1/3与中1/3交点（图39）。

【主治】头顶痛，眩晕，目昏花，咽喉痛，舌干，失音，小便不利，大便艰，小儿惊风，足心热，昏厥。

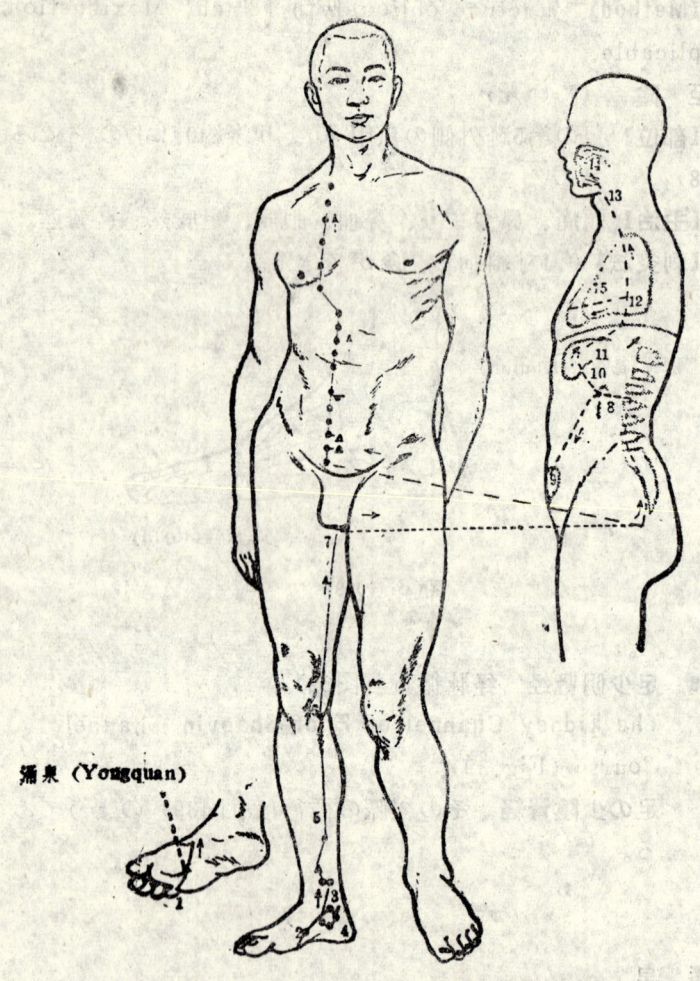

图(Fig.)39 足少阴肾经循行示意图
(The Kidney Channel of Foot-Shaoyin)

【刺灸法】直刺0.3～0.5寸；可灸。

Yongquan

【Location】In the depression appearing on the sole

when the foot is in plantar flexion, approximately at the junction of the anterior and middle third of the sole (Fig.39).

【Indications】 Pain in the vertex, dizziness, blurring of vision, sore throat, dryness of the tongue, aphonia, dysuria, dyschesia, infantile convulsion, feverish sensation in the sole, loss of consciousness.

【Method】 Puncture perpendicularly 0.3～0.5 inch. Moxibustion is applicable

湧泉 （ゆうせん）

【部位】土踏まずにあり、足を曲げ、指を曲げた時できる陥凹部の真中にある。足底の中心線上で、前から3分の1のところ。（図39）。

【主治】頭頂痛、眩暈、咽喉痛、舌が乾き、失語、小便が通じない。大便困難、小児驚風、足底熱、昏迷。

【刺灸法】0.3～0.5寸直刺し、灸ができる。

太 溪

【位置】内踝与跟腱之间凹陷中，平对内踝高点（图40）。

【主治】咽喉痛，齿痛，耳聋，咳血，气喘，月经不调，失眠，遗精，阳痿，小便频数，腰脊痛。

【刺灸法】直刺0.3寸；可灸。

Taixi

【Location】 In the depression between the medial malleolus and tendo calcaneus, level with the tip of the medial malleolus (Fig.40).

【Indications】Sore throat, toothache, deafness, hemoptysis, asthma, irregular menstruation, insomnia, seminal emission, impotence, frequency of micturition, pain in the lower back.

【Method】Puncture perpendicularly 0.3 inch. Moxibustion is applicable.

太　谿　（たいけい）

【部位】内踝とアキレス腱の間の陥凹部、内踝隆起と同じ水平線上にある（図40）。

【主治】咽喉痛、歯痛、難聴、咳血、喘息、月経不順、不眠、遺精、陰萎、頻尿、腰脊痛。

【刺灸法】0.3寸直刺し、灸ができる。

照　海

【位置】在内踝下1寸处（图40）。

【主治】月经不调，阴挺，阴痒，疝气，小便频数，痫证，咽喉干痛，失眠。

【刺灸法】直刺0.3～0.5寸；可灸。

Zhaohai

【Location】1 cun below the medial malleolus (Fig. 40).

【Indications】Irregular menstruation, prolapse of uterus, pruritus vulvae, hernia, frequency of micturition, epilepsy, sore throat, insomnia.

【Method】Puncture perpendicularly 0.3～0.5 inch. Moxibustion is applicable.

照　海（しょうかい）

【部位】内踝下1寸のところにある（図40）。
【主治】月経不順、子宮脱垂、陰部搔痒感、脱腸、頻尿、ひきつけ、咽喉が乾き、痛み、不眠。
【刺灸法】0.3～0.5寸直刺し、灸ができる。

复 溜

【位置】太溪直上2寸，当跟腱之前缘（图40）。
【主治】泄泻，肠鸣，水肿，腹胀，腿肿，足痿，盗汗，自汗。
【刺灸法】直刺0.3～0.5寸；可灸。
Fuliu
【Location】2 cun directly above Taixi, on the anterior border of tendo calcaneus (Fig.40).
【Indications】Diarrhea, borborygmus, edema, abdominal distension, swelling of leg, muscular atrophy, weakness and paralysis of foot, night sweeting, spontaneous sweating.
【Method】Puncture perpendicularly 0.3～0.5 inch. Moxibustion is applicable.
復 溜 （ふくりゅう）
【部位】太谿の直上2寸にあり、アキレス腱の前縁にあたる（図40）。
【主治】下痢、腸鳴、水腫、腹脹、腿腫、下肢の筋肉萎縮、寝汗、自汗。
【刺灸法】0.3～0.5寸直刺し、灸ができる。

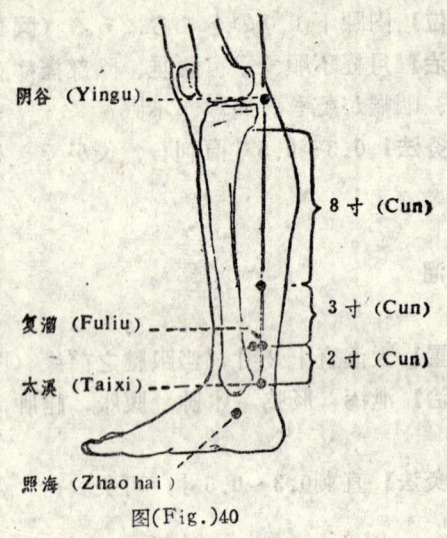
图(Fig.)40

9. **手厥阴心包经** 经脉循行（图41）。
The Pericardium Channel of Hand-Jueyin
Channel Course (Fig.41).
手の厥陰心包経　その経脈の循行は（図41）のようである。

間　使

【位置】在腕横纹上3寸，掌长肌腱与桡侧腕屈肌腱中间（图42）。
【主治】心痛，心悸，胃痛，呕吐，热病，烦躁，疟疾，癫狂，痫证，腋肿，肘挛，臂痛。
【刺灸法】直刺0.5～1寸；可灸。

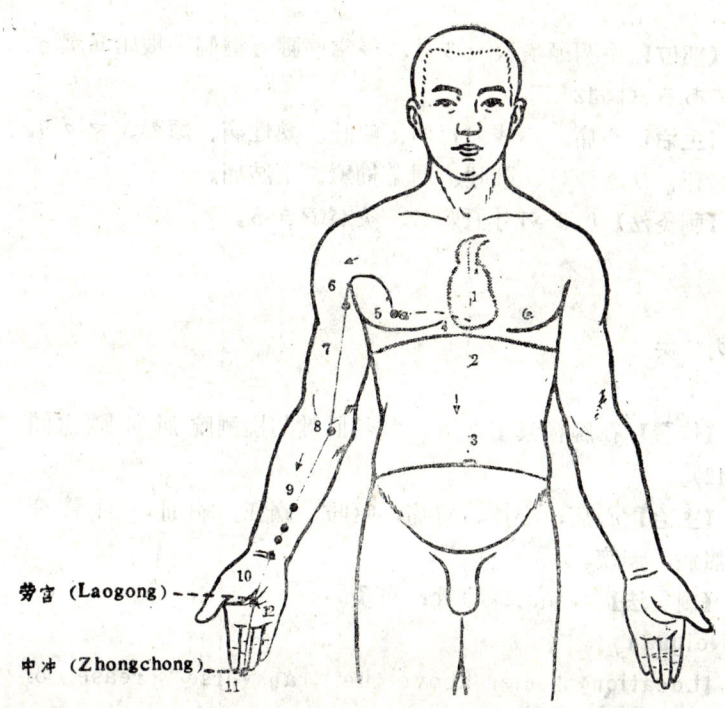

图(Fig.)41 手厥阴心包经循行示意图
(The Pericardium Channel of Hand-Jueyin)

Jianshi

【Location】 3 cun above the transverse crease of the wrist, between the tendons of m. palmaris longus and m. flexor carpi radialis (Fig. 42).

【Indications】 Cardiac pain, palpitation, gastric pain, vomiting, febrile diseases, irritability, malaria, mental disorders, epilepsy, swelling of the axilla, twitching or contracture of the elbow, pain of the arm.

【Method】 Puncture perpendicularly 0.5～1.0 inch. Moxibustion is applicable.

間 使 (かんし)

【部位】手関節横紋上3寸、長掌筋腱と橈側手根屈筋腱との間にある（図42）。

【主治】心痛、心悸、胃痛、嘔吐、熱性病、煩躁、マラリヤ、癲狂、ひきつけ、腋腫、肘部拘攣、上肢痛。

【刺灸法】0.5～1寸直刺し、灸ができる。

内　关

【位置】在腕横纹上2寸，掌长肌腱与桡侧腕屈肌腱之间（图42）。

【主治】心痛，心悸，胃痛，呕吐，癫狂，痫证，肘臂挛痛，热病，疟疾。

【刺灸法】直刺0.5～1寸；可灸。

Neiguan

[Location] 2 cun above the transverse crease of the wrist, between the tendons of m. palmaris longus and m.flexor carpi radialis (Fig.42).

[Indications] Cardiac pain, palpitation, gastric pain, vomiting, mental disorders, epilepsy, contracture and pain of the elbow and arm, febrile diseases, malaria.

[Method] Puncture perpendicularly 0.5～1.0 inch. Moxibustion is applicable.

内　関　（ないかん）

【部位】手関節横紋上2寸、長掌筋腱と橈側手根屈筋腱との間にある（図42）。

【主治】心痛、心悸、胃痛、嘔吐、癲狂，ひきつけ、上肢拘攣と痛み、熱性病、マラリヤ。

【刺灸法】0.5～1寸直刺し、灸ができる。

劳 宫

【位置】仰掌，在第2、3掌指关节之后的掌骨间，偏于第3掌骨桡侧（图41）。

【主治】心痛，癫狂，痫证，呕吐，口疮，口臭，鹅掌风。

【刺灸法】直刺0.3～0.5寸；可灸。

Laogong

[Location] When the hand is placed with the palm upward, the point is between the 2nd and 3rd metacarpal bones, proximal to the metacarpophalangeal joint, on the radial side of the 3rd metacarpal bone(Fig.41).

[Indications] Cardiac pain, mental disorders, epilepsy, vomiting, stomatitis, foul breath, fungus infection of hand and foot.

[Method] Puncture perpendicularly 0.3～0.5 inch. Moxibustion is applicable.

労 宮 （ろうきゅう）

【部位】手掌を上にして、第2、3中手指関節後の中手骨間、第3中手骨の橈側にかたよる（図41）。

【主治】心痛、癲狂、ひきつけ、嘔吐、口腔潰瘍、口臭、手癬。

【刺灸法】0.3～0.5寸直刺し、灸ができる。

中 冲

【位置】在手中指尖端之中央处（图41）。

【主治】心痛，烦闷，昏厥，舌强不语，热病，中暑，惊

厥，掌中热。

【刺灸法】斜刺0.1寸，或三棱针点刺出血；可灸。

Zhongchong

【Location】 In the centre of the tip of the middle finger(Fig. 41).

【Indications】 Cardiac pain, irritability, syncope aphasia with stiffness of the tongue, febrile diseases, heat stroke, convulsion, feverish sensation in the palm.

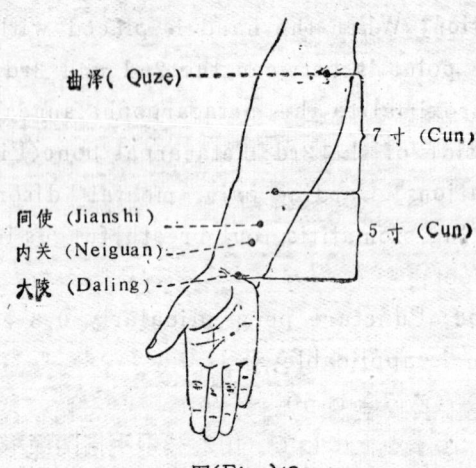

图(Fig.)42

【Method】 Puncture obliquely 0.1 inch, or prick with three-edged needle to cause bleeding. Moxibustion is applicable.

中　衝　（ちゅうしょう）

【部位】中指先の中央にある。

【主治】心痛、煩悶、昏迷、舌強、熱性病、日射病、驚厥、手掌熱（図41）。

【刺灸法】0.1寸斜刺し、あるいは三稜針で点刺して出血

させる。灸ができる。

10. 手少阳三焦经　经脉循行（图43）。
The Sanjiao Channel of Hand-Shaoyang
Channel Course (Fig.43).
手の少陽三焦経　その経脈の循行は（図43）のようである。

中渚

【位置】俯掌，在手背第4、5掌骨间，掌指关节后方凹陷处（图44）。
【主治】头痛，目赤，耳聋，耳鸣，咽喉肿痛，肘臂痛，手指不能屈伸，热病。
【刺灸法】直刺0.3～0.5寸；可灸。
Zhongzhu
[Location] When the hand is placed with the palm facing downward, the point is on the dorsum of hand between the 4th and 5th metacarpal bones, in the depression proximal to the metacarpophalangeal joint (Fig. 44).
[Indications] Headache, redness of the eyes, deafness, tinnitus, sore throat, pain in the elbow and arm, motor impairment of fingers, febrile diseases.
[Method] Puncture perpendicularly 0.3～0.5 inch. Moxibustion is applicable.
中渚　（ちゅうしょ）

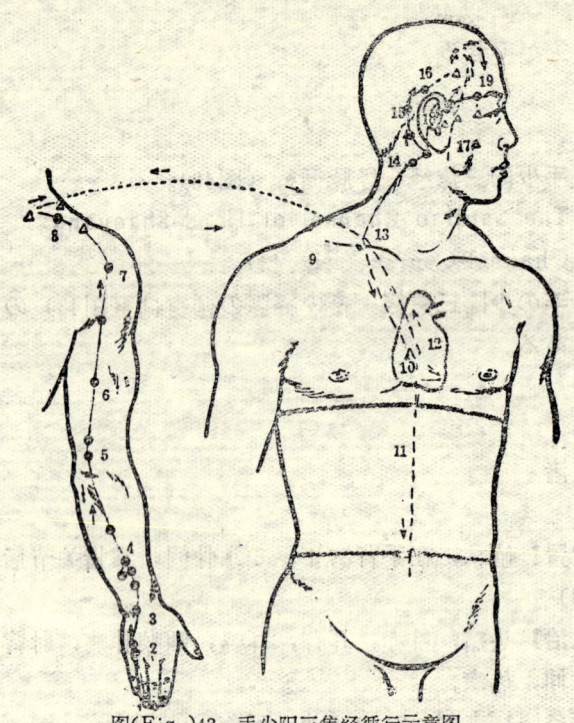

図(Fig.)43 手少阳三焦经循行示意图
(The Sanjiao Channel of Hand-Shaoyang)

【部位】手掌を下にして、手背の第4、5中手骨間、中手指関節後方の陥凹にある（図44）。

【主治】頭痛、目赤、難聴、耳鳴、咽喉腫痛、上肢痛、指の屈伸不便、熱性病。

【刺灸法】0.3～0.5寸直刺し、灸ができる。

外 关

【位置】在阳池上2寸（阳池在尺腕关节部指总伸肌腱尺侧凹陷处)当尺、桡两骨间（图44）。

【主治】热病，头痛，颊痛，胁痛，耳聋，耳鸣，肘臂屈伸不利，手指痛，手颤。

【刺灸法】直刺0.7～1寸；可灸。

Waiguan

[Location] 2 cun above Yangchi, which is at the junction of the ulna and carpal bones, in the depression lateral to the tendon of m. extensor digitorum communis, between the radius and ulna (Fig. 44).

[Indications] Febrile diseases, headache, pain in the cheek and the hypochondriac region, deafness, tinnitus, motor impairment of the elbow and arm, pain of fingers, hand tremor.

[Method] Puncture perpendicularly 0.7～1.0 inch. Moxibustion is applicable.

外　関　（がいかん）

【部位】陽池の上2寸（陽池は尺骨手根関節部、総指伸筋腱の尺側の陥凹したところにある）尺骨・橈骨間にある（図44）。

【主治】熱性病、頭痛、顔面痛、側胸痛、難聴、耳鳴、上肢伸展不便、指痛、手震顫。

【刺灸法】0.7～1寸直刺し、灸ができる。

支　沟

【位置】在阳池上3寸，尺、桡两骨之间（图44）。

【主治】暴瘖，耳鸣，耳聋，肩背酸重，呕吐，便秘。

【刺灸法】直刺0.7～1寸；可灸。

Zhigou

[Location] 3 cun above Yangchi, between the ulna and radius (Fig. 44).

【Indications】Sudden hoarseness of voice, tinnitus, deafness, aching and heavy sensation of the shoulder and back, vomiting, constipation.

【Method】Puncture perpendicularly 0.7~1.0 inch. Moxibustion is applicable.

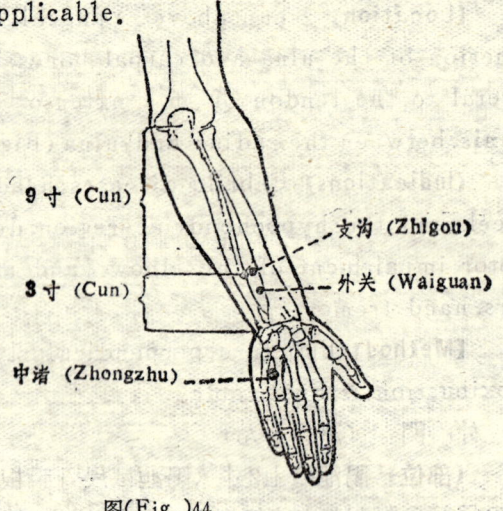

图(Fig.)44

支　溝　（しこう）
　【部位】陽池の上3寸、尺、橈骨間にある（図44）。
　【主治】急発性の失音（話す時に聲がでない）、耳鳴、難聴、肩こり、嘔吐、便秘。
　【刺灸法】0.7～1寸直刺し、灸ができる。

翳风

　【位置】耳垂后，下颌角与乳突之间凹陷中（图45）。
　【主治】耳鸣，耳聋，口眼歪斜，牙关紧闭，颊肿。
　【刺灸法】直刺0.5～1寸；可灸。

Yifeng

【Location】 Posterior to the lobule of the ear, in the depression between the mandible and mastoid process (Fig.45).

【Indications】 Tinnitus, deafness, facial paralysis, trismus, swelling of the cheek.

【Method】 Puncture perpendicularly 0.5～1.0 inch. Moxibustion is applicable.

翳風　（えいふう）

【部位】耳垂後、下顎角と乳様突起の間の陥凹したところにある（図45）。

【主治】耳鳴、難聴、口と目の歪み、歯が閉じ、顔面腫。

【刺灸法】0.5～1寸直刺し、灸ができる。

耳　門

【位置】在耳屏上切迹之前方与下颌髁状突稍上方之凹陷处，张口取穴（图45）。

【主治】耳聋，耳鸣，聤耳，齿痛。

【刺灸法】直刺0.3～0.5寸；可灸。

Ermen

【Location】 In the depression anterior to the supratragic notch and slightly superior to the condyloid process of the mandible. The point is located with the mouth open(Fig.45).

【Indications】 Deafness, tinnitus, otorrhea, toothache.

【Method】 Puncture perpendicularly 0.3～0.5 inch. Moxibustion is applicable.

耳　門　（じもん）
【部位】上耳珠切痕の前方と下顎髁状突起上方の陥凹したところ，口をあけて取る（図45）。
【主治】難聴、耳鳴、耳だれ、歯痛。
【刺灸法】0.3～0.5寸直刺し、灸ができる。

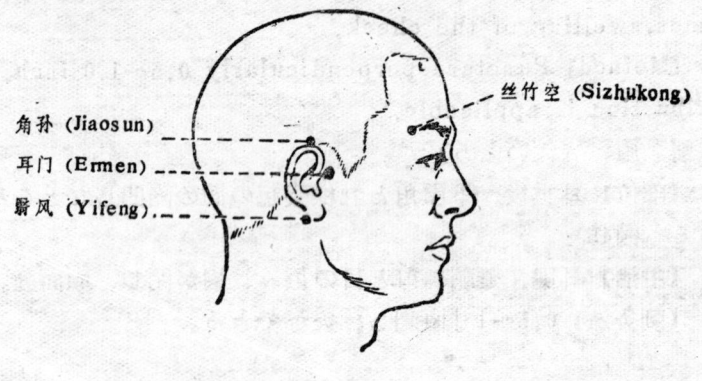

图(Fig.)45

11. 足少阳胆经　经脉循行（图46）。
The Gall Bladder Channel of Foot-Shaoyang
Channel Course(Fig.46).
足の少陽胆経　その経脈の循行は（図46）のようである。

瞳子髎

【位置】在目外眦外方，眶骨外側縁凹陥中（図47）。
【主治】头痛，目痛，视力减退，目赤流泪。
【刺灸法】向外方沿皮刺0.2～0.3寸；可灸。

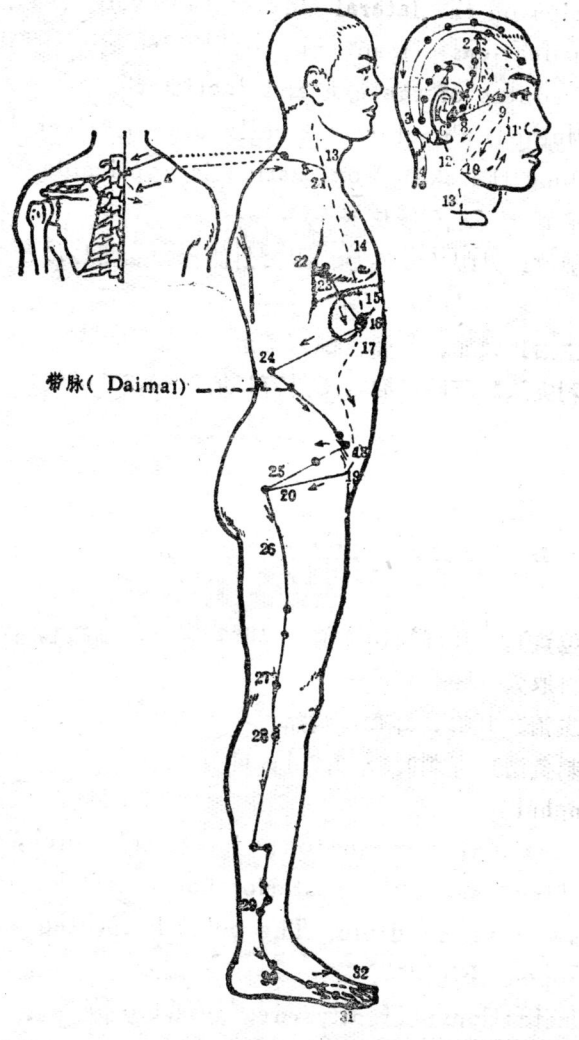

图(Fig.)46 足少阳胆经循行示意图
(The Gall Bladder Channel of Foot-Shaoyang)

Tongziliao

【Location】 Lateral to the outer canthus, in the depression on the lateral side of the orbit (Fig.47).

【Indications】 Headache, ophthalmalgia, failing of vision, redness of the eye and lacrimation.

【Method】 Puncture laterally 0.2～0.3 inch horizontally along the skin. Moxibustion is applicable.

瞳子髎　（どうしりょう）

【部位】外眼角の外方、眼窩外側縁の陥凹したところ（図47）。

【主治】頭痛、眼痛、視力減退、目赤、流涙。

【刺灸法】皮膚に沿って外方に0.2～0.3寸横刺し、灸ができる。

听会

【位置】在耳屏间切迹前，当听宫直下，下颌髁状突之后缘，张口取穴（图47）。

【主治】耳鸣，耳聋，齿痛。

【刺灸法】直刺0.5～0.7寸；可灸。

Tinghui

【Location】 Anterior to the intertragic notch, directly below Tinggong, at the posterior border of the condyloid process of the mandible. The point is located with the mouth open (Fig.47).

【Indications】 Tinnitus, deafness, toothache.

【Method】 Puncture perpendicularly 0.5～0.7 inch. Moxibustion is applicable.

聴　会　（ちょうえ）
【部位】珠間切痕の前、聴宮穴の直下方、下顎小頭の後縁にある。口を開いて取穴する（図47）。
【主治】耳鳴、難聴、歯痛。
【刺灸法】0.5～0.7寸直刺し、灸ができる。

阳　白

【位置】在前额眉毛中央上1寸，约当前发际与眉毛之间上2/3与下1/3交点（图47）。
【主治】前额痛，目眩，迎风流泪，外眦疼痛，眼睑瞤动。
【刺灸法】向下沿皮刺0.3～0.5寸；可灸。

Yangbai

【Location】On the forehead, 1 cun above the midpoint of the eyebrow, approximately at the junction of the upper two-thirds and lower third of the vertical line drawn from the anterior hairline to the eyebrow (Fig.47).

【Indications】Frontal headache, blurring of vision, lacrimation on exposure to wind, pain in the outer canthus, twitching of eyelids.

【Method】Puncture 0.3～0.5 inch horizontally along the skin with the needle directed downward. Moxibustion is applicable.

陽　白　（ようはく）
【部位】前額の眉毛中央の上方約1寸のところ、前髪の生際と眉毛との間上の2/3と下の1/3の交叉点にある（図47）。
【主治】前額痛、目眩、流涙、外眼角痛、眼瞼痙攣。

【刺灸法】皮膚に沿って下向きに0.3〜0.5寸刺し、灸ができる。

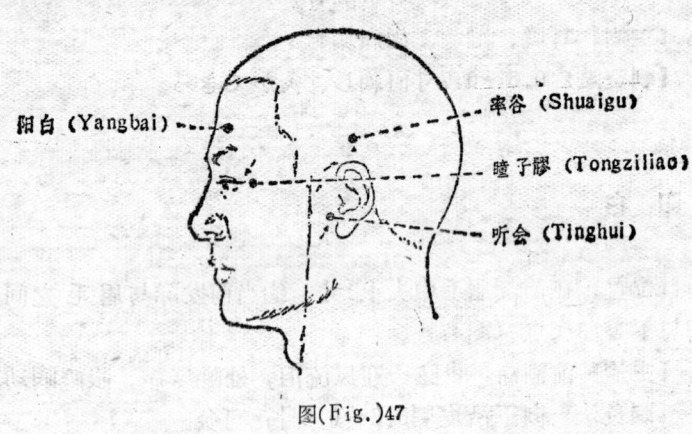

图(Fig.)47

风　池

【位置】在项后，枕骨下，当胸锁乳突肌与斜方肌上端之间凹陷处（图48）。

【主治】头痛，眩晕，颈项强痛，目赤痛，鼻渊，肩背痛，热病，感冒。

【刺灸法】向鼻尖方向直刺0.5〜1寸；可灸。

Fengchi

[Location] In the posterior aspect of the neck, below the occipital bone, in the depression between the upper portion of m. sternocleidomastoideus and m. trapezius (Fig.48).

[Indications] Headache, dizziness, pain and stiffness of the neck, red and painful eyes, rhinorrhea, pain in the shoulder and back, febrile diseases, common cold.

[Method] Puncture perpendicularly 0.5〜1.0 inch towards the tip of the nose. Moxibustion is applicable.

風 池 （ふうち）

【部位】後頭骨隆起直下の陷凹したところと乳様突起との間、僧帽筋と胸鎖乳様筋上端との間にある（図48）。

【主治】頭痛、眩暈、頸項部強直痛、結膜炎、鼻ポリープ、肩背痛、熱性病、感冒。

【刺灸法】鼻尖に向かって0.5〜1寸直刺し、灸ができる。

带 脉

【位置】在第11肋端直下，与脐相平处（图46）。

【主治】月经不调，带下，疝气，腰胁痛。

【刺灸法】直刺0.5〜1寸；可灸。

Daimai

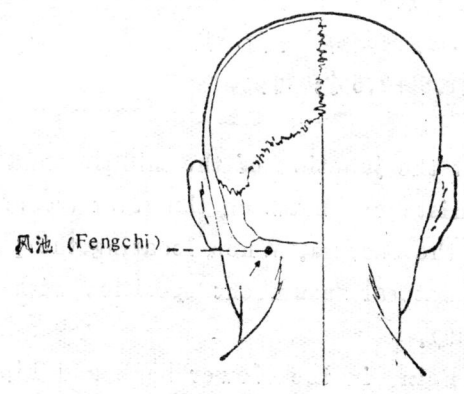

図(Fig.)48

【Location】 Directly below the free end of the 11th rib, level with the umbilicus (Fig. 46).

【Indications】 Irregular menstruation, leukorrhea, hernia, pain in the lower back and hypochondriac region.

【Method】 Puncture perpendicularly 0.5～1.0 inch. Moxibustion is applicable.

帯脈 （たいみゃく）

【部位】第11肋骨端（章門穴）の直下、臍と水平線上にある（図46）。

【主治】月経不順、腰痛、帯下、ヘルニア、季肋部痛。

【刺灸法】0.5～1寸直刺し、灸ができる。

环跳

【位置】在股骨大转子与骶管裂孔的连线上，中1/3与外1/3交点，侧卧屈股取穴（图49）。

【主治】腰胯痛，下肢痿痹，半身不遂。

【刺灸法】直刺1.5～2.5寸；可灸。

Huantiao

【Location】 At the junction of the middle and lateral third of the distance between the great trochanter and the hiatus of the sacrum. When locating the point, put the patient in lateral recumbent position with the thigh flexed (Fig. 49).

【Indications】 Pain in the lower back and hip region, muscular atrophy, motor impairment, pain and weakness of the lower extremities, hemiplegia.

【Method】 Puncture perpendicularly 1.5～2.5 inches. Moxibustion is applicable

環　跳　（かんちょう）

【部位】側臥位させて（下腿を伸展し、大腿を屈曲する）大腿骨大転子最高点と仙骨裂孔との連結線上の中1/3と外1/3の交叉点にある（図49）。

【主治】腰痛、下肢麻痺、半身不遂。

【刺灸法】1.5～2.5寸直刺し、灸ができる。

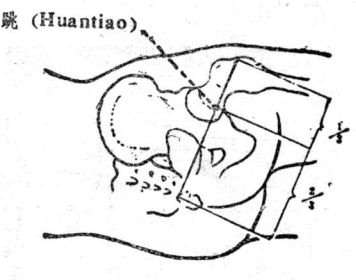

図(Fig.)49

风　市

【位置】在大腿外侧中线上，腘横纹上7寸；直立垂手时，约当中指尖所点处（图50）。

【主治】半身不遂，下肢痿痹、麻木，遍身瘙痒。

【刺灸法】直刺0.7～1.2寸；可灸。

Fengshi

【Location】On the midline of the lateral aspect of the thigh, 7 cun above the transverse politeal crease. When the patient is standing erect with the hands close to the sides, the point is where the tip of the middle finger touches (Fig. 50).

【Indications】Hemiplegia, muscular atrophy, motor impairment and pain of the lower extremities, general pruritus.

【Method】 Puncture perpendicularly 0.7～1.2 inches Moxibustion is applicable.

風市 （ふうし）

【部位】大腿外側の中線の上、膝膕横紋の上7寸のとこ

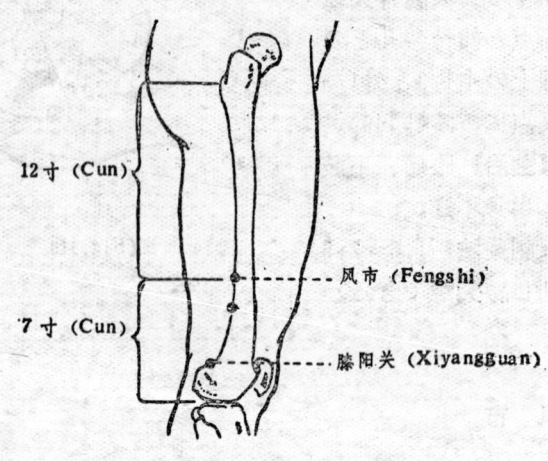

図(Fig.)50

ろ。直立して上肢を下げ、その中指の尖端があたるところ（図50）。

【主治】半身不遂、下肢麻痺、しびれ、全身搔痒感。

【刺灸法】0.7～1.2寸直刺し、灸ができる。

阳陵泉

【位置】在腓骨小头之前下方凹陷处（图51）。

【主治】半身不遂，下肢痿、痹、麻木，膝肿痛，胁肋痛，口苦，呕吐。

【刺灸法】直刺0.8～1.2寸；可灸。

Yanglingquan

[Loation] In the depression anterior and inferior to the head of the fibula(Fig.51).

[Indications] Hemiplegia, muscular atrophy, motor impairment, numbness and pain of the lower extremities, pain and swelling of the knee, pain in the hypochondriac and costal region, bitter taste in mouth, vomiting.

[Method] Puncture perpendicularly 0.8～1.2 inches. Moxibustion is applicable.

陽陵泉　（ようりょうせん）

【部位】腓骨頭の前下方の陥凹したところにある（図51）。

【主治】半身不遂、下肢萎縮、麻痺、膝腫脹痛、側胸痛、口が苦い、嘔吐。

【刺灸法】0.8～1.2寸直刺し、灸ができる。

悬　钟（又名绝骨）

【位置】在外踝高点上3寸，当腓骨后缘与腓骨长、短肌肌腱之间凹陷处（图51）。

【主治】半身不遂，颈项强，胸腹胀满，胁痛，膝腿痛，脚气。

【刺灸法】直刺0.4～0.5寸；可灸。

Xuanzhong (Also known as Juegu)

[Location] 3 cun above the tip of the external malleolus, in the depression between the posterior border of the fibula and the tendons of m. peronaeus longus and brevis (Fig.51).

【Inodications】 Hemiplegia, neck rigidity, fullness of the chest, distension of the abdomen, pain in the hypochondriac region, knee and leg, beriberi.

【Method】 Puncture perpendicularly 0.4～0.5 inch. Moxibustion is applicable.

懸　鐘　（けんしょう）（ぜっこつともいう）

【部位】外踝隆起の上3寸、腓骨後縁、長腓骨筋と短腓骨筋との間の陥凹したところにある（図51）。

【主治】半身不遂、頸項部強直、胸腹膨満、脇痛、下肢疼痛、脚気。

【刺灸法】0.4～0.5寸直刺し、灸ができる。

足窍阴

【位置】在第4趾外侧，趾甲角后1分许（图51）。
【主治】偏头痛，目痛，耳聋，胁痛，多梦，热病。
【刺灸法】斜针0.1～0.2寸；可灸。

Foot-Qiaoyin

【Location】 On the lateral side of the 4th toe, about 0.1 cun posterior to the corner of the nail (Fig.51).

【Inodications】 One-sided headache, ophthalmalgia, deafness, pain in the hypochondriac region, dream-disturbed sleep, febrile diseases.

【Method】 Puncture obliquely 0.1～0.2 inch. Moxibustion is applicable.

足竅陰　（あしきょういん）

【部位】第4趾の外側、爪甲根部より0.1寸のところ（図51）。

【主治】側頭痛、目痛、難聴、脇痛、多夢、熱性病。

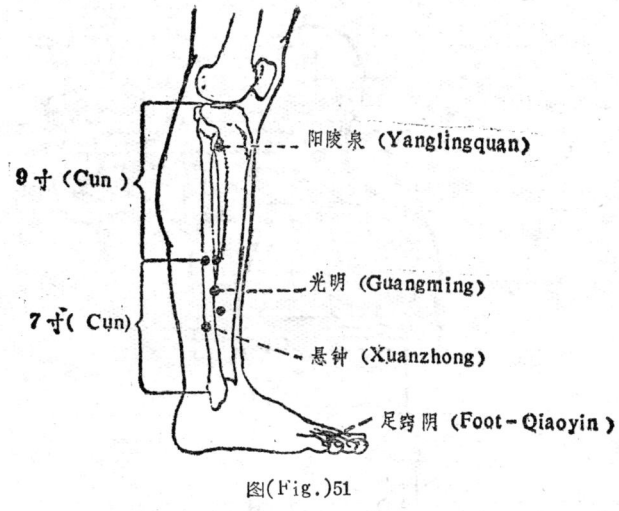
図(Fig.)51

【刺灸法】0.1〜0.2寸斜刺し、灸ができる。

12. 足厥阴肝经　经脉循行（图52）。
The Liver Channel of Foot-Jueyin
Channel Course (Fig.52).
足の厥陰肝経　その経脈の循行は（図52）のようである。

行　間

【位置】在足第1、2趾的趾缝间，趾蹼缘之后方（图53）。
【主治】月经过多，尿道疼痛，遗尿，小便不通，疝气，口角歪斜，目赤肿痛，胁痛，头痛，目眩，痫证，抽搐，失眠。
【刺灸法】斜刺0.5寸；可灸。

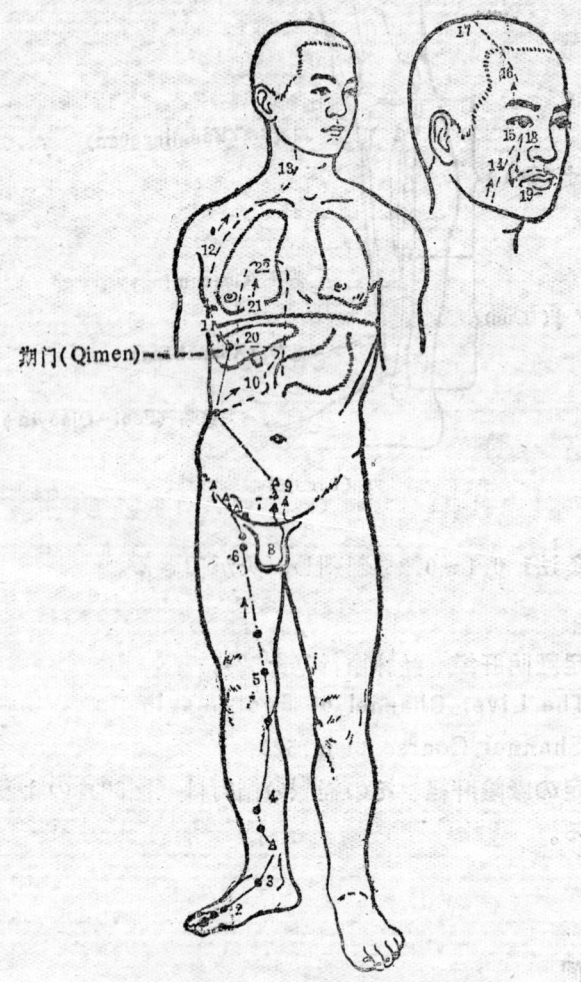

图(Fig.)52 足厥阴肝经循行示意图
(The Liver Channel of Foot-Jueyin)

Xingjian

〖Location〗 Between the 1st and 2nd toe, proximal to the margin of the web (Fig.53).

【Indications】 Menorrhagia, urethralgia, enuresis, retention of urine, hernia, deviation of mouth, redness, swelling and pain of the eye, pain in the hypochondriac region, headache, blurring of vision, epilepsy, convulsion, insomnia.

【Method】 Puncture obliquely 0.5 inch. Moxibustion is applicable.

行　間　（こうかん）

【部位】足の第1、第2指の間隙、指の付根の後方0.5寸のところ（図53）。

【主治】月経過多、尿道疼痛、遺尿、尿閉、ヘルニア、口の歪み、結膜炎、脇痛、頭痛、目眩、ひきつけ、搐搦、不眠。

【刺灸法】0.5寸斜刺し、灸ができる。

太　冲

【位置】在第1、2跖骨结合部之前凹陷中（图53）。

【主治】崩漏，疝气，遺尿，小便不通，內踝前缘痛，胁胀，口角歪斜，小儿惊风，痫证，头痛，眩晕，失眠。

【刺灸法】直刺0.5寸；可灸。

Taichong

【Location】 In the depression distal to the junction of the 1st and 2nd metatarsal bones (Fig.53).

【Indications】 Uterine bleeding, hernia, enuresis, retention of urine, pain in the anterior aspect of the medial malleolus, fullness in the hypochondriac region, deviation of mouth, infantile convulsion, epilepsy, headache, vertigo, insomnia.

【Method】Puncture perpendicularly 0.5 inch. Moxibustion is applicable.

太衝 （たいしょう）

【部位】足の第1、第2中足指関節の間の陥凹したところ（図53）。

【主治】崩漏、ヘルニア、遺尿、尿閉、内踝前縁痛、脇部脹満、口の歪み、小児搐搦、癲癇、頭痛、眩暈、不眠。

【刺灸法】0.5寸直刺し、灸ができる。

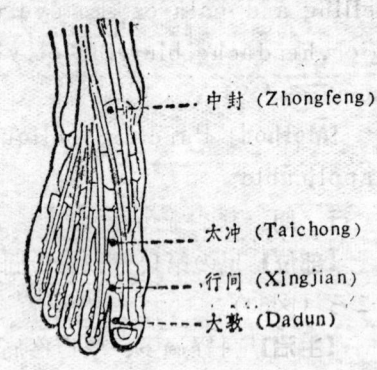

图(Fig.)53

期　门

【位置】在乳中线上，乳头下2肋间，当第6肋间隙（图52）。

【主治】胸胁疼痛，腹胀，胸满，呕吐，呃逆。

【刺灸法】斜刺0.3寸；可灸。

Qimen

【Location】On the mammillary line, two ribs below the nipple, in the 6th intercostal space (Fig.52).

【Indications】Pain in the chest and hypochondriac region, abdominal distension, fullness of the chest, vomiting, hiccup.

【Method】Puncture obliquely 0.3 inch. Moxibustion is applicable.

期　門　（きもん）

【部位】乳中線上、乳頭の下方2肋間目にあり、第6、7肋間隙にある（図52）。

【主治】側胸部疼痛、腹脹、胸悶、嘔吐、吃逆。

【刺灸法】0.3寸斜刺し、灸ができる。

13．督脉　经脉循行（图54）。

The Du Channel　Channel Course (Fig.54).

督脈　のそ経脈の循行は（図54）のようである。

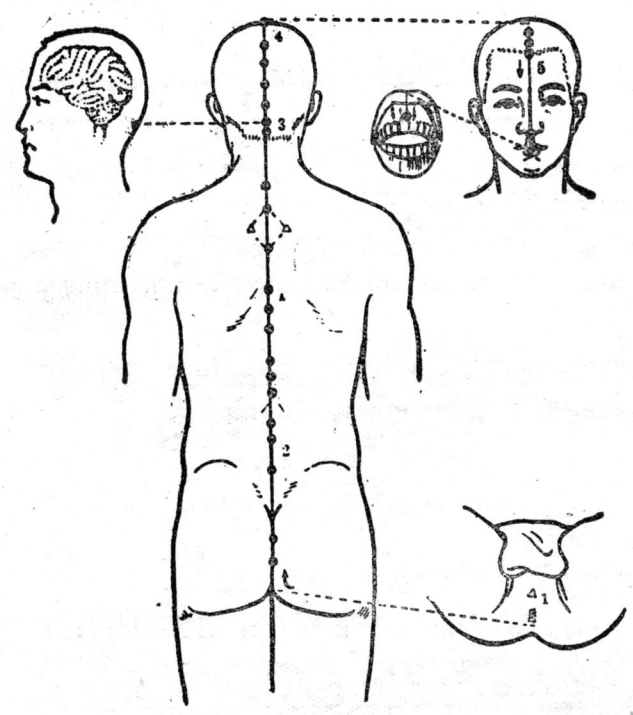

图(Fig.)54　督脉循行示意图
(The Du Channel)

长　强

【位置】在尾骨尖端与肛门之间的中点，伏卧取穴（图55）。
【主治】便血，泄泻，便秘，痔疾，脱肛，腰脊痛。
【刺灸法】直刺0.5～1寸；可灸。

Changqiang

〖Location〗 Midway between the tip of the coccyx and the anus. Locate the point in prone position (Fig. 55).

〖Indications〗 bloody stool, diarrhea, constipation, hemorrhoids, prolapse of rectum, pain in the lower back.

〖Method〗 Puncture perpendicularly 0.5～1.0 inch. Moxibustion is applicable.

長　強　（ちょうきょう）

【部位】尾骨先と肛門との間の中点にあり、伏臥位で取る（図55）。
【主治】血便、下痢、便秘、痔疾、脱肛、腰脊痛。
【刺灸法】0.5～1寸直刺し、灸ができる。

命　門

【位置】在第2腰椎棘突下（图55）。
【主治】脊强，腰痛，带下，阳痿，遗精，泄泻。
【刺灸法】直刺0.5～1寸；可灸。

Mingmen

〖Location〗 Below the spinous process of the 2nd lumbar vertebra (Fig. 55).

【Indications】 Stiffness of the back, lumbago, leukorrhea, impotence, seminal emission, diarrhea.

【Method】 Puncture perpendicularly 0.5～1.0 inch. Moxibustion is applicable.

命　門　（めいもん）

【部位】第2腰椎棘突起の下にある（図55）。

【主治】脊柱強直、腰痛、白帯下、陰萎、遺精、下痢。

【刺灸法】0.5～1寸直刺し、灸ができる。

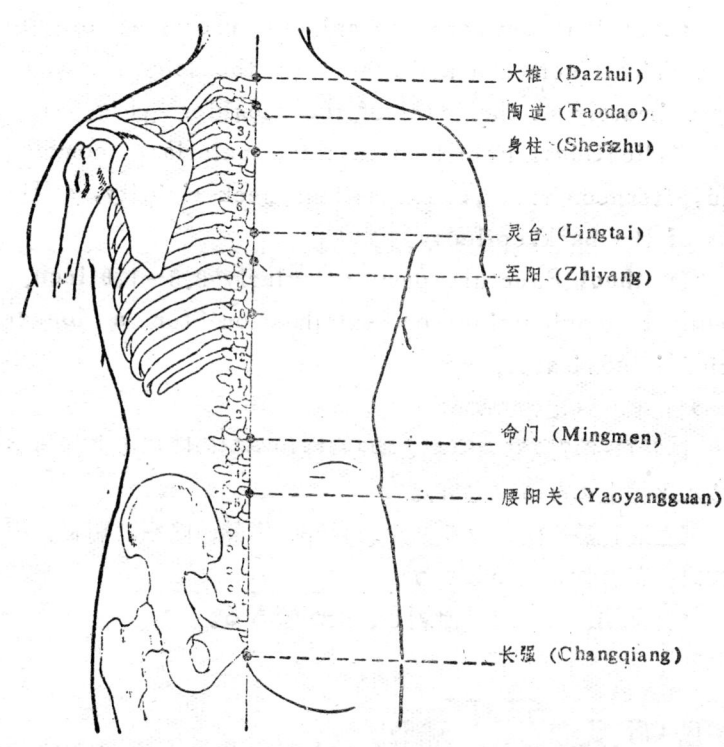

図(Fig.)55

大　椎

【位置】在第7颈椎棘突与第1胸椎棘突之间，约与肩相平（图55）。

【主治】热病，疟疾，感冒，骨蒸潮热，咳嗽，气喘，项强，脊背强急，痫证。

【刺灸法】直刺0.5～1寸；可多灸。

Dazhui

【Location】Between the spinous processes of the 7th cervical vertebra and the 1 st thoracic vertebra, approximately at the level of the shoulder (Fig.55).

【Indications】Febrile diseases, malaria, common cold, afternoon fever, cough, asthma, neck rigidity, stiffness of the back, epilepsy.

【Method】Puncture perpendicularly 0.5～1.0 inch. Frequent moxibustion or moxibustion for a longer period is advisable.

大　椎　（だいつい）

【部位】第7頸椎棘突起と第1胸椎棘突起の間にあり、肩と同じ水平線上にある（図55）。

【主治】熱性病、マラリヤ、風邪、潮熱、咳嗽、喘息、項部強直、背脊強直、ひきつけ。

【刺灸法】0.5～1寸直刺し、灸ができる。

風　府

【位置】在枕骨粗隆直下，两侧斜方肌之间的凹陷中取之

（图56）。

【主治】头痛，项强，目眩，鼻衄，咽喉肿痛，中风不语，癫狂，半身不遂。

【刺灸法】直刺0.5～1寸，不宜深刺。

Fengfu

〖Location〗 Directly below the external occipital protuberance, in the depression between m. trapezius of both sides (Fig.56).

〖Indications〗 Headache, neck rigidity, blurring of vision, epistaxis, sore throat, post-apoplexy aphasia, mental disorders, hemiplegia.

〖Method〗 Puncture perpendicularly 0.5～1.0 inch. Deep puncture is not advisable.

風　府　（ふうふ）

【部位】外後頭隆起の直下、両側斜方筋の間の陥凹のところ（図56）。

【主治】頭痛、項部強直、目眩、鼻血、咽喉腫痛、卒中失語、癲狂、半身不遂。

【刺灸法】0.5～1寸直刺し、深く刺してはいけない。

百　会

【位置】后发际上7寸，约当两侧耳廓尖连线之中点取之（图56）。

【主治】癫狂，中风，头痛，头晕，耳鸣，目眩，鼻塞，脱肛。

【刺灸法】沿皮刺0.3～0.5寸；可灸。

Baihui

[Location] 7 cun above the posterior hairline, on the midpoint of the line connecting the apexes of the two auricles(Fig.56).

[Indications] Mental disorders, apoplexy, headache, dizziness, tinnitus, blurring of vision, nasal obstruction, prolapse of rectum.

[Method] Puncture 0.3〜0.5 inch horizontally along the skin. Moxibustion is applicable.

百　会　（ひゃくえ）

【部位】後髪生際の上7寸、両側耳介最高点の連結線上の中点に取る（図56）。

【主治】癲狂、卒中、頭痛、眩暈、耳鳴、目眩、鼻つまり、脱肛。

【刺灸法】皮膚に沿って0.3〜0.5寸刺し、灸ができる。

上　星

【位置】入前发际1寸，百会前4寸（图56）。

【主治】头痛，目痛，鼻渊，鼻衄，癫狂。

【刺灸法】向后沿皮刺0.3〜0.5寸，或用三棱针点刺出血；可灸。

Shangxing

[Location] 1 cun within the anterior hairline, 4 cun anterior to Baihui (Fig.56).

[Indications] Headache, ophthalmalgia, rhinorrhea, epistaxis, mental disorders.

[Method] Puncture 0.3〜0.5 inch posteriorly horizontally along the skin, or prick with three-edged needle to cause bleeding. Moxibustion may be applied.

上星　（じょうせい）

【部位】前髪際から1寸、百会の前4寸（図56）。

【主治】頭痛、目痛、鼻竇炎（蓄膿症）、鼻血、癲狂。

【刺灸法】皮膚に沿って後向き0.3～0.5寸刺す。或は三稜針で点刺して瀉血する。灸ができる。

人　中　（又名水沟）

【位置】在鼻柱下，人中沟近上方正中（图56）。

【主治】癫狂，痫证，小儿惊风，昏迷，牙关紧闭，口眼歪斜，面肿，腰脊强痛。

【刺灸法】向上斜刺0.2～0.3寸。

Renzhong (Also Known as Shuigou)

〖Location〗 Below the nose, a little above the midpoint of the philtrum (Fig. 56).

〖Indications〗 Mental disorders, epilepsy, infantile

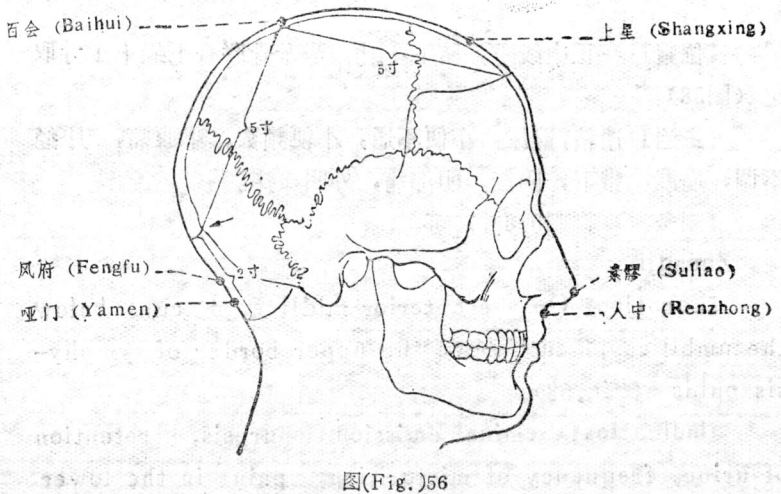

图(Fig.)56

convulsion, coma, trismus, facial paralysis, swelling of the face, pain and stiffness of the lower back.

【Method】 Puncture obliquely upward 0.2~0.3 inch.

人中　（にんちゅう）（すいこうともいう）

【部位】鼻柱の下、人中溝の上から3分の1のところの真中（図56）。

【主治】癲狂、搐搦、小児ひきつけ、昏迷、歯をくいしばる、口と目の歪み、顔面腫、腰脊強痛。

【刺灸法】0.2～0.3寸上に向け斜刺する。

14. 任脉　经脉循行（图57）。
The Ren Channel　Channel Course (Fig.57).
任脈　その経脈の循行は（図57）のようである。

中极

【位置】在正中线上，脐下4寸，当耻骨联合上缘上1寸取之（图58）。

【主治】遗精，遗尿，小便不通，小便频数，小腹痛，月经不调，崩漏，带下，阴挺，阴部痛，外阴瘙痒。

【刺灸法】直刺0.8寸；可灸。

Zhongji

【Location】 On the anterior midline, 4 cun below the umbilicus, 1 cun above the upper border of symphysis pubis (Fig.58).

【Indicatios】 Seminal emission, enuresis, retention of urine, frequency of micturition, pain in the lower

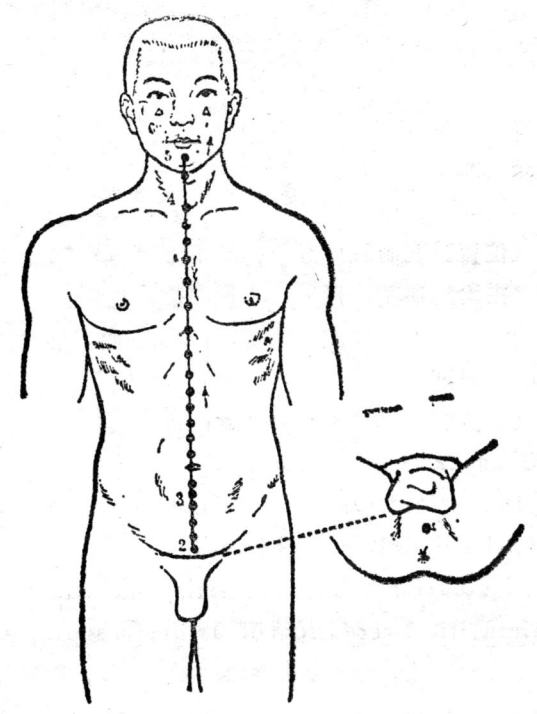

図(Fig.)57 任脈循行示意図
(The Ren Channel)

abdomen, irregular menstruation, uterine bleeding, leukorrhea, prolapse of uterus, pain of the external genitalia, pruritus vulvae.

【Method】 Puncture perpendicularly 0.8 inch. Moxibustion is applicable.

中　極　（ちゅうきょく）

【部位】腹正中線上、臍下4寸にあり、恥骨結合上縁の上1寸に取る（図58）。

【主治】遺精、遺尿、排尿困難、頻尿、下腹痛、月経不

順、月経過多、白帯下、子宮脱出、生殖器痛、陰部搔痒感。
【刺灸法】0.8寸直刺し、灸ができる。

关　元

【位置】在腹正中线上，脐下3寸（图58）。
【主治】遗精，遗尿，小便频数，小便不通，月经不调，痛经，闭经，带下，崩漏，阴挺，产后出血，疝气，小腹痛，泄泻，中风脱证。
【刺灸法】直刺0.8～1.2寸；可多灸。
Guanyuan
【Location】On the midline of the abdomen, 3 cun below the umbilicus (Fig.58).
【Indications】Seminal emission, enuresis, frequency of micturition, retention of urine, irregular menstruation, dysmenorrhea, amenorrhea, leukorrhea, uterine bleeding, prolapse of uterus, postpartum hemorrhage, hernia, lower abdominal pain, diarrhea, flaccid type of apoplexy.
【Method】Puncture perpendicularly 0.8～1.2 inches. Moxibustion may be applied fairly long and frequently.
関　元　（かんげん）
【部位】腹正中線上、臍の下3寸（図58）。
【主治】遺精、遺尿、頻尿、尿閉、月経不順、月経痛、無月経、白帯下、月経過多、子宮脱出、産後出血、ヘルニア、下腹痛、下痢、卒中の脱症。
【刺灸法】0.8～1寸直刺し、灸が多くできる。

气　海

【位置】在腹正中线上，脐下1.5寸（图58）。

【主治】崩漏，带下，月经不调，产后出血，疝气，遗尿，腹痛，泄泻，便秘，水肿，中风脱证。

【刺灸法】直刺0.8～1.2寸；可多灸。

Qihai

【Location】On the midline of the abdomen, 1.5 cun below the umbilicus (Fig.58).

【Indications】Uterine bleeding, leukorrhea, irregular menstruation, postpartum hemorrhage, hernia, enuresis, abdominal pain, diarrhea, constipation, edema, flaccid type of apoplexy.

【Method】Puncture perpendicularly 0.8～1.2 inches. Moxibustion may be applied often.

気　海　（きかい）

【部位】腹正中線上、臍の下1.5寸（図58）。

【主治】月経過多、白帯下、月経不順、産後出血、ヘルニア、遺尿、腹痛、下痢、便秘、水腫、卒中の脱症。

【刺灸法】0.8～1.2寸直刺し、灸が多くできる。

中　脘

【位置】在腹正中线上，脐上4寸（图58）。

【主治】胃痛，腹胀，翻胃吞酸，呕吐，泄泻，痢疾，完谷不化。

【刺灸法】直刺1～1.5寸；可灸。

Zhongwan

— 133 —

【Location】On the midline of the abdomen, 4 cun above the umbilicus(Fig.58).

【Indications】Gastric pain, abdominal distension, regurgitation, vomiting, diarrhea, dysentery, stool with undigested food.

【Method】Puncture perpendicularly 1.0～1.5 inches. Moxibustion is applicable.

中脘 （ちゅうかん）

【部位】腹正中線上、臍の上4寸（図58）。

【主治】胃痛、腹脹、呑酸、嘔吐、赤痢、下痢、消化不良。

【刺灸法】1～1.5寸直刺し、灸ができる。

膻中

【位置】在胸骨正中线上，两乳头之间，平第4肋间隙（图58）。

【主治】气喘，呃逆，胸痛，产妇乳汁少。

【刺灸法】沿皮刺0.3～0.5寸；可灸。

Shanzhong

【Location】On the midline of the sternum, between the nipples, level with the 4th intercostal space (Fig. 58).

【Indications】Asthma, hiccup, pain in the chest, lactation deficiency.

【Method】Puncture 0.3～0.5 inch horizontally along the skin. Moxibustion is applicable.

膻中 （だんちゅう）

【部位】胸骨正中線上、両乳頭の間、第4肋骨間隙と同じ

水平線上にある（図58）。

【主治】喘息、しゃっくり、胸痛、乳汁分泌不足。

【刺灸法】皮膚に沿って0.3～0.5寸刺す。灸ができる。

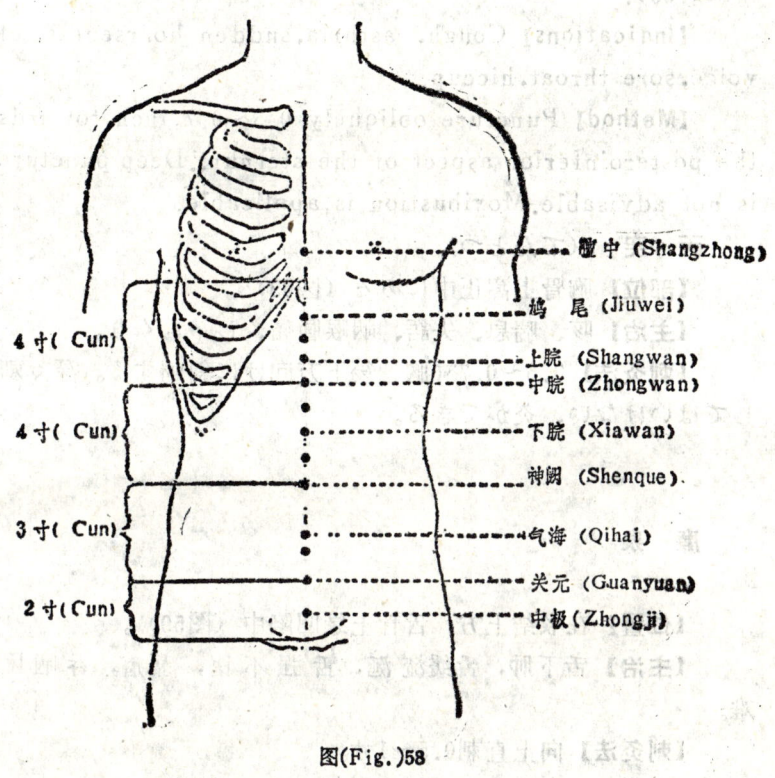

図(Fig.)58

天　突

【位置】在胸骨上窩正中（図59）。

【主治】咳嗽，气喘，暴瘖，咽喉肿痛，呃逆。

【刺灸法】向胸骨后下方斜刺0.5～0.7寸，不宜深刺；可

灸。

Tiantu

【Location】In the centre of the suprasternal fossa (Fig.59).

【Indications】Cough, asthma, sudden hoarseness of voice, sore throat, hiccup.

【Method】Puncture obliquely 0.5〜0.7 inch towards the posteroinferior aspect of the sternum. Deep puncture is not advisable. Moxibustion is applicable.

天　突　（てんとつ）

【部位】胸骨上窩正中にある（図59）。

【主治】咳、喘息、失語、咽喉腫痛、しゃっくり。

【刺灸法】0.5〜0.7寸胸骨後下方向けに斜刺する。深く刺してはいけない、灸ができる。

廉　泉

【位置】在喉结上方，舌骨上缘凹陷中（图59）。

【主治】舌下肿，舌缓流涎，舌强不语，暴瘖，吞咽困难。

【刺灸法】向上直刺0.5〜1寸。

Lianquan

【Location】Above the Adam's apple, in the depression at the upper border of the hyoid bone (Fig.59).

【Indications】Swelling of the subglossal region, salivation with glossoplegia, aphasia with stiffness of tongue, sudden hoarseness of voice, difficulty in swallowing.

【Method】Puncture perpendicularly 0.5～1.0 inch with the needle directed upward.
廉　泉　（れんせん）
【部位】喉頭隆起の上方、舌骨上縁の陥凹にある（図59）。
【主治】舌下腫、流涎、舌強直、失語、嗄声、嚥下困難。
【刺灸法】0.5～1寸、上に向け直刺する。

承　浆

【位置】在颏唇沟正中凹陷处（图59）。
【主治】口眼歪斜，面肿，龈肿，齿痛，流涎，癫狂。
【刺灸法】向上斜刺0.2～0.3寸；可灸。
Chengjiang
【Location】In the depression in the centre of the mentolabial groove (Fig.59).
【Indications】Facial paralysis, facial swelling, swelling of the gums, toothache, salivation, mental disorders.
【Method】Puncture obliquely upward 0.2～0.3 inch. Moxibustion is applicable.
承　浆　（しょうしょう）
【部位】オトガイ唇溝正中の陥凹にある（図59）。
【主治】顔面神経麻痺、顔面腫、歯齦腫、歯痛、流涎、癲狂。
【刺灸法】0.2～0.3寸上に向け斜刺し、灸ができる。

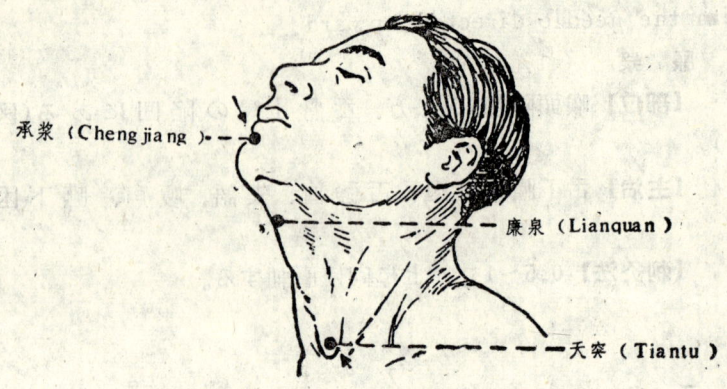

图(Fig.)59

15. 经外奇穴
Extraordinary Points
经外奇穴

四神聪

【位置】在百会前后左右各1寸（图60）。
【主治】头痛，眩晕，失眠，健忘，痫证。
【刺灸法】斜刺0.5～1寸。

Sishencong

【Location】A group of 4 points at the vertex, 1 cun respectively posterior, anterior, and lateral to Baihui (Fig.60).

【Indications】Headache, dizziness, insomnia, poor memory, epilepsy.

【Method】Puncture obliquely 0.5～1.0 inch.

四神聡　（ししんそう）

【部位】百会の前、後、左、右それぞれ1寸のところ（図60）。
【主治】頭痛、眩暈、不眠、健忘、ひきつけ。
【刺灸法】0.5～1寸斜刺する。

印　堂

【位置】在两侧眉头连线之中点（图60）。
【主治】小儿惊风，前额痛，鼻渊。
【刺灸法】向下方沿皮刺0.3～0.5寸，或点刺出血。

Yintang

【Location】Midway between the medial ends of the two eyebrows (Fig.60).
【Indications】Infantile convulsion, frontal headache, rhinorrhea.
【Method】Puncture 0.3～0.5 inch downward horizontally along the skin, or prick to cause bleeding.

印　堂　（いんどう）

【部位】眉間の中点にある（図60）。
【主治】小児ひきつけ、前頭痛、鼻竇炎（蓄膿症）。
【刺灸法】下に向け皮膚に沿って0.3～0.5寸刺し、あるいは点刺して瀉血する。

太　陽

【位置】在眉梢与目外眦连线之中点，向后约1寸处凹陷中（图60）。

— 139 —

【主治】头痛，目赤肿痛。
【刺灸法】直刺或向后斜刺0.3～0.4寸，或用三棱针点刺出血。

Taiyang

【Location】In the depression about 1 cun posterior to the midpoint between the lateral end of the eyebrow and the outer canthus (Fig.60).

【Indications】Headache, redness, swelling and pain of the eye.

【Method】Puncture perpendicularly or obliquely and posteriorly 0.3～0.4 inch, or prick with three-edged needle to cause bleeding.

太 陽 （たいよう）

【部位】まゆげの外端と外眼角の連線の中点から後へ約1寸の陥凹にある（図60）。

【主治】頭痛、目赤腫痛。

【刺灸法】0.3～0.4直刺し、あるいは後へ向け斜刺し、または三稜針で点刺して瀉血する。

金津　玉液

【位置】在舌下系带两侧静脉上（图61）。

【主治】呕吐不止，舌强不语。

【刺灸法】舌尖舐着上腭，在舌根部静脉上，用三棱针点刺出血。

Jinjin Yuye

【Location】On the veins on both sides of the frenulum of the tongue (Fig.61).

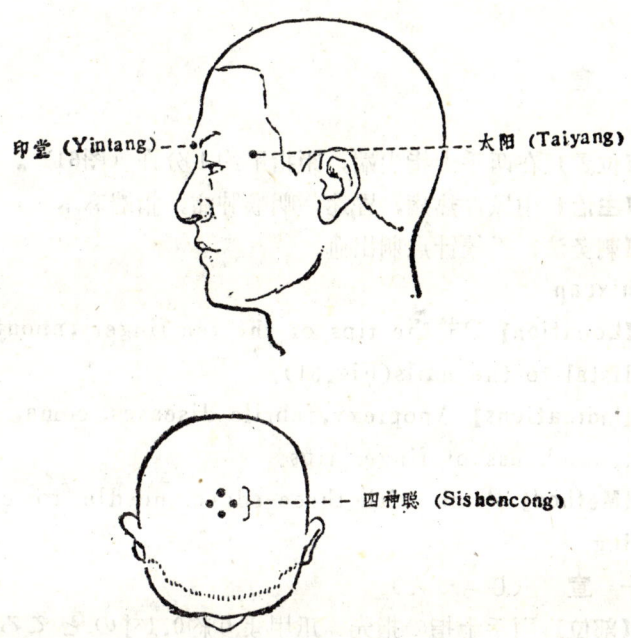

图(Fig.)60

【Indications】 Continual vomiting, aphasia with stiffness of tongue.

【Method】 Ask the patient to place the tip of the tongue on the hard palate. Prick the veins with three-edged needle to cause bleeding.

金津　玉液（きんしん、ぎょくえき）

【部位】舌小帯両側の静脈にある。（図61）。

【主治】嘔吐止まらず、舌強失語。

【刺灸法】舌尖を硬口蓋にあて、舌根の静脈に三稜針で点刺して瀉血する。

— 141 —

十 宣

【位置】在两手十指尖端，距指甲约1分许（图61）。
【主治】中风，热病，昏迷，咽喉肿痛，指端麻木。
【刺灸法】三棱针点刺出血。
Shixuan

[Location] On the tips of the ten fingers, about 0.1 cun distal to the nails(Fig.61).

[Indications] Apoplexy, febrile diseases, coma, sore throat, numbness of finger tips.

[Method] Prick with three-edged needle to cause bleeding.

十 宣 （じっせん）

【部位】両手十指の指先、爪甲より約0.1寸のところ（図61）。
【主治】卒中、熱性病、昏迷、咽喉腫痛、指のしびれ。
【刺灸法】三稜針で点刺して瀉血する。

华佗夹脊

【位置】从第1胸椎至第5腰椎，每椎沿棘突旁边各一穴。相传为华佗取背俞法（图62）。
【主治】与背俞穴相类似。上背部夹脊穴，主胸部、心、肺病证；下背部夹脊穴，主上腹部、肝、胆、脾、胃病证；腰部夹脊穴，主下腹部、肾、肠、膀胱及下肢病证。
【刺灸法】沿棘突旁边直刺，胸椎部0.5～1寸；腰椎部1.5

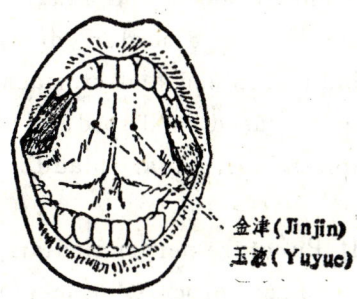
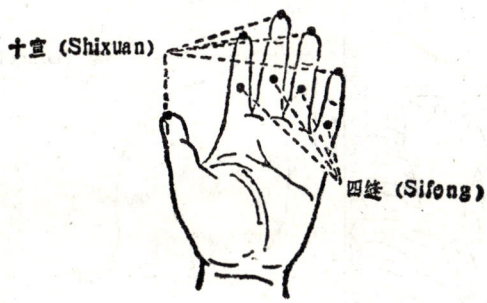

图(Fig.)61

~2寸；均可灸。

Huatuo Jiaji

【Location】 A group of points on both sides of the spinal column at the lateral borders of each spinous process from the 1st thoracic vertebra to the 5th lumbar vertebra. It is believed that these points were used as Back-Shu Points by the ancient famous doctor Huatuo (Fig. 62).

【Indications】 Similar to those of Back-Shu Points.

The Jiaji Points on the upper back are indicated in disorder of the chest, heart and lung; those on the lower back are indicated in disorder of the upper abdomen, liver, gall bladder, spleen and stomach; and those in the lumbar region are used in disorder of the lower abdomen, kidney, intestines, urinary bladder and lower extremities.

【Method】 Puncture perpendicularly along the lateral side of the spinous process, 0.5~1.0 inch for points

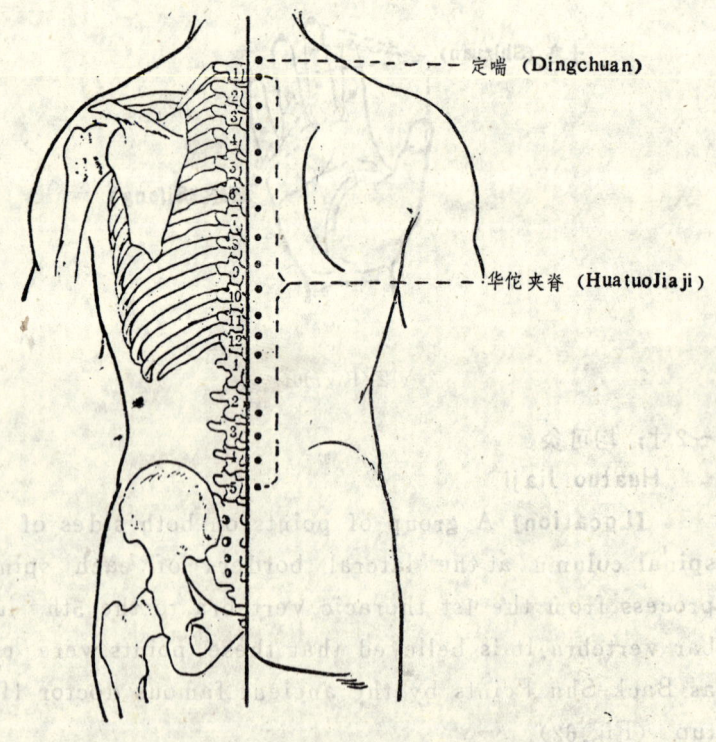

图(Fig.)62

along the thoracic vertebrae and 1.5～2.0 inches for those along the lumbar vertebrae. Moxibustion is applicable.

華佗夾脊（かだきょうせき）

【部位】第1胸椎から第5腰椎まで、椎骨ごとに棘突起の傍にそれぞれ一穴ある。華佗が背兪を取る方法であるといわれている（図62）。

【主治】背兪穴に似ている。背の上部の夾脊穴は、胸部、心、肺病症を主り、背の下部の夾脊穴は、上腹部、胆、肝、脾、胃の病症を主り、腰部の夾脊穴は、下腹部、腎、腸、膀胱及び下肢の病症を主る。

【刺灸法】棘突起の傍に沿って直刺する。胸椎部は0.5～1寸。腰椎部は1.5～2寸で宜しい、みな灸ができる。

中篇　针灸的临床治疗

PART B　Clinical Therapy of Acupuncture and Moxibustion

中篇　針灸の臨床治療

中篇　針灸的臨床治療

PART B Clinical Therapy of
Acupuncture and Moxibustion

中篇　針灸の臨床治療

第五章 处方配穴的基本原则

针灸是"从外治内"的,针灸体表的腧穴,运用补虚泻实等方法,可以治疗各种病证。针灸处方配穴,以循经取穴为基本原则,这是根据经络的循行、腧穴的分布及其主治性能而决定的,具体有三方面。

Chapter V The Basic Principles Governing Prescription and Combination of Points

Acupuncture and moxibustion are methods of "treating diseases of the interior from the exterior". Various diseases may be cured by the application of methods for reinforcing the deficiency, and reducing the excess, by using the points of the body surface. The basic principle for prescribing and combining points is to select points according to the course of the channel, the distribution of points and their indications. There are three ways of selecting points in clinical practice.

第五章　処方配穴の基本原則

　針灸は従外治内（体外で治療を施して体内の病気を治す）のものである。体表の腧穴に針刺あるいは灸を施して、虚であれば補法を、実であれば瀉法を用いるなどの方法で、いろいろな病気を治療することができる。針灸の処方配穴は、循経取穴（経脈に沿って穴位を取る）を基本的原則とする。すなわち、病がどの経絡と関係があるかを判断して、関係ある経絡のツボを治療に用いる。したがって、経絡の循行ルート、腧穴の分布及びその経脈の主治効能などをよく理解しなければならない。具体的な応用については、次の三つの方法がある。

　1．远道取穴　当诊断病变属于哪一经络、哪一脏腑之后，取其有关经络的四肢部有关腧穴，即是远道取穴。例如：脘腹部疾患取足三里，面部疾患取合谷等。远道取穴还包括"上病下取"和"下病上取"两种治疗方法。"上病下取"以肘、膝以下的腧穴为主，如颈项痛取后溪；"下病上取"，如久痢脱肛取百会，腰脊痛取人中等。

　1. Selection of Remote Points　After the involved channel and organ are determined, points below the elbow or knee of the involved channel are selected. For instance, Zusanli is chosen to treat gastric or abdominal disorders; Hegu may be punctured for diseases of the face, etc. Selection of remote points also includes choosing points on the lower part of the body to treat diseases of the upper part, and vice versa. This is essentially to select points below the elbow and knee as the principal ones. For neck pain, for instance, Houxi is chosen; An example of selecting points on the upper part of the body to treat a disease of the lower part is the selection of Baihui to treat prolapse of the rectum due to chronic dysentery, and Renzhong to treat low back pain, etc.

1. 遠隔取穴 病状がどの経絡、どの臟腑に属するかをまず診察したのち、関係ある経絡の四肢、遠隔部位に位置する腧穴を取穴して治療する方法である。例えば、腹部の疾患には足三里を、顔面部の疾患には合谷を取るなどは、その例である。また遠隔取穴は、上病下取（疾患が上部にある場合、下部の穴位を取る）、下病上取（疾患が下部にある場合、上部の穴位を取る）という二つの方法を含む。上病下取は、主として肘、膝以下の腧穴を取る。例えば、頸項部痛では後谿を取るなどである。下病上取は、例えば、久しく下痢して脱肛になった場合、百会を取り、腰、背部の痛みには人中を取るなどである。

2. 局部取穴 在病痛的局部取穴即是局部取穴。例如：头痛取上星，胃痛取中脘等。

2. Selection of Local Points The selection of the points in a local pain area is known as the selection of local points. For example, Shangxing is chosen to treat headache, Zhongwan to treat gastric pain, etc.

2. 局部取穴 病痛の局部で穴位を選ぶ方法を局部取穴という。例えば、胃痛なら中脘を、頭痛なら上星を取るなどである。

3. 邻近取穴 在病痛的邻近部选取腧穴，即是邻近取穴。例如：胃脘痛取章门，目疾取风池等。本法可配合局部取穴以加强疗效，也可代替局部取穴。

3. Selection of Adjacent Points Selecting points in the adjacent area to the area of pain is known as the selection of adjacent points. For instance, Zhangmen is used to treat gastric pain, Fengchi is used in deseases of the eye. For strengthening the therapeutic effect local points may be combined with adjacent points, or adjacent points can substitute for local points.

3. 近処取穴 病痛に近い部位で穴位を取る方法は近処取穴である。例えば、胃痛に章門を、目の疾患に風池を取るなどはその例である。この方法は局部取穴とくみあわせることにより、治療の効果を高めることができる。局部取穴のかわりにこの方法をとってもよい。

以上三种取穴法，可以单独应用，也可配合应用。例如：胃脘痛于远道取足三里、内关，局部取中脘或邻近取章门等。

对肢体两侧的病证，还可结合"左病取右，右病取左"的交叉取穴法。例如：口眼歪斜，半身不遂等证，在患侧取穴，也可在健侧取穴；又如：右牙痛取左合谷，左牙痛取右合谷等。

The above three methods of selecting points may be used separately or in combination. For instance the selection of Zusanli and Neiguan in the remote area combined with Zhongwan in the local area or Zhangmen in the neighbouring area may be considered for treating gastric pain.

The crossing methods of selecting points may also be used i.e. selecting points on the right side to treat disorders of the left, and vice versa. For instance, points may be chosen on the affected side or the healthy side to treat facial paralysis or hemiplegia. Hegu of the right hand may be punctured for toothache on the left side, and vice versa.

　以上の三種類の配穴方法は、単獨に使っても、くみあわせて使ってもよい。例えば、胃痛に、遠隔取穴では足三里、内関を取り、局部取穴では中脘を取り、近処取穴では章門を取るなどがその例である。

　また、肢体の両側の病症に対しては、左病取右（左側の病症は右側の穴位を取る）、右病取左（右側の病症は左側の穴位を取る）という左右交叉の取穴方法を使ってもよい。例えば、顔面神経麻痺、半身麻痺などの病症に、患側の穴位を使ってもよいし、健側の穴位を取ってもよい。また右側の歯痛には左側の合谷を取り、左側の歯痛には右側の合谷を取るなどがその例である。

第六章　常见病证的针灸治疗

Chapter Ⅵ　Treatment of Common Diseases with Acupuncture and Moxibustion

第六章　よく見かける病症の針灸治療

感　冒

【辨证】

风寒：恶寒发热无汗，头痛，鼻塞，流涕，肢节酸痛，或兼咽痒咳嗽，舌苔薄白，脉浮紧。

风热：发热，恶风，汗出，头胀，口干喉燥，咽部发红或痛，舌苔薄黄，脉浮数。

【治疗】

处方：

风寒：外关、风池、列缺、合谷。

风热：大椎、风池、曲池、合谷。

随证配穴：头痛：太阳；鼻塞：迎香。

　　　　　预防感冒：在本病流行季节，可每日灸风池、足三里，有一定预防作用。

The Common Cold

【Differentiation】

Common cold due to wind-cold: Chills, fever, anhidrosis, headache, nasal obstruction, rhinitis, aching of joints. There may be the complication of itching of the throat, and cough. Fur of tongue is thin and white, the pulse superficial and tense.

Common cold due to wind-heat: Fever, intolerance to wind, hidrosis, distending sensation of head, thirst, hacking cough, dry, congested and sore throat, thin and yellowish tongue coating, superficial and rapid pulse.

【Treatment】

Prescription:
Wind-cold: Waiguan, Fengchi, Lieque, Hegu.
Wind-heat: Dazhui, Fengchi, Quchi, Hegu.
Points according to symptoms and signs:
Headache: Taiyang.
Nasal obstruction: Yingxiang.
Prophylaxis:
Application of moxibustion to Fengchi or Zusanli daily may prevent the common cold when this disease is prevalent.

感　冒

【弁症】

風寒によるもの：発熱、悪寒、無汗、頭痛、鼻づまり、鼻

水。四肢の関節がだるく、あるいは咽部の搔痒感、咳嗽など種種の症状が見られる。舌苔は薄白で、脈は浮緊である。

風熱によるもの：発熱、悪風、汗が出て、頭が重い。口が乾いて喉部の津液がなくなり、咽喉部は充血、あるいは痛む。舌苔は薄黄で、脈は浮数である。

【治療】

処方：

風寒によるもの：外関、風池、列缺、合谷。

風熱によるもの：大椎、風池、曲池、合谷。

症状による配穴：頭痛：太陽。鼻づまり：迎香。

感冒の予防：本病の流行シーズンに毎日風門あるいは足三里に灸を施せば、ある程度の予防作用がある。

咳　　嗽

【辨证】

外感：

风寒：恶寒发热，头痛，鼻塞，咳嗽不畅，苔薄白，脉浮。

风热：发热，口渴，不恶寒，咳嗽，痰黄稠，苔黄，脉浮而数。

内伤：

肺燥阴虚：干咳无痰或痰少，咽喉干燥或疼，或痰中带血丝甚至咯血，潮热，颧红，舌红苔薄，脉虚数。

脾阳虚：咳嗽痰多，入冬更剧，饮食减少，精神不振，舌苔白滑厚腻，脉沉迟。

【治疗】

处方：

外感：列缺、合谷、肺俞、尺泽。风寒可针灸并用，风热则只针不灸。

内伤：

肺燥阴虚：肺俞、列缺、照海。

脾阳不振：脾俞、中脘、足三里、肺俞、丰隆。

Cough

【Differentiation】

Invasion of exogenous pathogenic factors:

Wind-cold type: Chills, fever, headache, nasal obstruction, choking cough. The tongue has a thin white coating, the pulse is superficial.

Wind-heat type: Fever without chills, thirst, cough with purulent thick sputum, tongue with yellowish coating, superficial rapid pulse.

Endogenous factors:

Dryness of the lung due to xu (deficiency) of yin: Dry cough with no or scanty sputum, dry or sore throat. There may be bloody sputum or even hemoptysis, afternoon fever, malar flush. Red tongue with thin coating, feeble rapid pulse.

Xu (Deficiency) of yang of spleen: Cough with excessive sputum which becomes severe in winter, anorexia, listlessness, thick sticky slippery white-coated tongue, pulse usually deep and slow.

【Treatment】

Prescription:

Invasion by exogenous pathogenic factors: Lieque, Hegu, Feishu, Chize. For wind-cold type, acupuncture may be combined with moxibustion, while for wind-heat type use acupuncture only.

Endogenous factors:

Dryness of the lung due to xu (deficiency) of yin: Feishu, Lieque, Zhaohai.

Xu (deficiency) of yang of spleen: Pishu, Zhongwan, Zusanli, Feishu, Fenglong.

咳　嗽

【弁症】

外感によるもの：

風寒：悪寒、発熱、頭痛、鼻づまり、咳が出にくい。舌苔は薄白で、脈は浮である。

風熱：発熱、口渇、悪寒なく、咳があって痰は粘稠で黄色。舌苔は黄色で、脈は浮数である。

内傷によるもの：

肺燥陰虚：乾咳無痰または痰が少ない、咽喉部乾燥感があるか痛みがある。あるいは痰に細い系状の血を帯び、甚だしきは喀血、潮熱、頬が赤くなる。舌質が赤く、舌苔が薄い。脈は虚数である。

脾陽虚：咳があって痰が多い。冬になるとひどくなる。食欲減退、精神不振。舌苔は白くなめらかで、しかも厚く粘り気がある。脈は多く沈遅である。

【治療】

処方：

外感によるもの：列缺、合谷、肺俞、尺沢。風寒の場合は針と灸を併用し、風熱の場合は針だけを用いる。

内傷によるもの：

　　肺燥陰虚：肺俞、列缺、照海。

　　脾陽不振：脾俞、中脘、足三里、肺俞、豊隆。

喘　証

【辨证】

实喘：

风寒：喘咳痰稀，气急，多兼发热恶寒，无汗等症，苔白，脉浮。

痰热：呼吸急促，声高气粗，胸闷，痰稠多黄，苔黄厚，脉滑数有力。

虚喘：

肺虚：呼吸短促，语言无力，动则易汗，脉虚弱等。

肾虚：动则喘作，气短不续，形寒肢冷，脉沉细无力等。

【治疗】

实喘：

风寒：肺俞、列缺、合谷。

痰热：丰隆、天突、尺泽、定喘。

虚喘：

肺虚：肺俞、太渊、足三里。

肾虚：肾俞、命门、气海、膻中。

随证配穴：脾虚：脾俞、中脘。

Asthma

【Differentiation】

Shi type:
Wind-cold: Cough with thin sputum, shortness of breath. Usually there are accompanying symptoms of fever, chills, anhidrosis, white coating on tongue, superficial pulse.

Phlegm-heat: Rapid and coarse breathing, stifling sensation in the chest, thick purulent sputum, thick yellowish coating on tongue, rapid, rolling and forceful pulse.

Xu type:
Xu of lung: Short and quick breathing, weak and low voice, hidrosis, weak pulse.

Xu of kidney: Asthma, dyspnea upon exertion, chilliness with cold extremities, deep thready feeble pulse.

【Treatment】

Prescription:
Shi type:
Wind-cold: Feishu, Lieque, Hegu.
Phlegm-heat: Fenglong, Tiantu, Chize, Dingchuan.
Xu type:
Xu of lung: Feishu, Taiyuan, Zusanli.
Xu of kidney: Shenshu, Mingmen, Qihai, Shanzhong.

Secondary points:
Xu of spleen: Pishu, Zhongwan.

喘　息

【弁症】

実喘:
風寒:喘息、咳があって痰が稀薄である。呼吸困難、多くは発熱、悪寒、無汗などの症状が同時に見られる。舌苔は白く、脈は浮である。
痰熱:呼吸促迫、聲が高く呼吸が粗い。胸悶、痰は粘稠で多くは黄色。舌苔は厚く黄色で、脈は滑数で力が強い。

虚喘:
肺虚:呼気が多く吸気が少ない。言語無力、動くと汗が出る。脈は虚弱である。
腎虚:動くと喘息がはげしくなり、呼吸が短促し、とぎれとぎれになるような感じになり、寒がり、手足が冷える。脈は沈細で力が弱い。

【治療】

実喘:
風寒:肺俞、列缺、合谷。
痰熱:豊隆、天突、尺沢、定喘。
虚喘:
肺虚:肺俞、太淵、足三里。
腎虚:腎俞、命門、気海、膻中。
症状による配穴:脾虚:脾俞、中脘。

中　暑

【辨证】

本病可分为轻、重两证：

轻证：头痛，汗多，皮肤灼热，气粗，舌燥，口干，烦渴，脉浮大而数。

重证：先见头痛，烦渴，呼吸喘急，继而突然昏倒，不省人事，汗出，脉沉而无力。

【治疗】

处方：

轻证：大椎、委中、合谷、曲池、金津、玉液。

重证：人中、百会、委中、十宣。

Sunstroke

[Differentiation]

Sunstroke may be divided into mild and severe types.

Mild type: Headache, hidrosis, hot skin, coarse breathing, dry tongue and mouth, thirst, superficial large and rapid pulse.

Severe type: Headache, thirst, fast short breathing followed by sudden collapse, loss of consciousness, sweating, deep and forceless pulse.

【Treatment】

Prescription:

Mild type: Dazhui, Weizhong, Hegu, Quchi, Jinjin, Yuye.

Severe type: Renzhong, Baihui, Weizhong, Shixuan.

日射病

【弁症】

本病は軽いものと重いものの二種類に分けられる。

　軽いもの：頭痛、汗が多く、皮膚に灼熱感があり、呼吸が粗く、舌が乾燥し、口が渇き、煩渇がある。脈は浮大で、しかも数である。

　重いもの：まず頭痛、煩渇、呼吸困難があって、さらに突然昏倒し、人事不省になり、汗が出る。脈は沈で、しかも無力である。

【治療】

処方：

軽いもの：大椎、委中、合谷、曲池、金津、玉液。

重いもの：人中、百会、委中、十宣。

呃　逆

【辨证】

　实证：多由食积，气滞，脘腹胀满，呃声洪亮，烦闷不舒，苔黄腻，脉滑实或弦有力。

虚寒证：呃声沉缓有力，得热则减，苔白润，脉迟缓。

【治疗】

处方：足三里、中脘、内关、膈俞、天突。
随证配穴：食积气滞：内庭、太冲。虚寒：上脘（灸）。

Hiccup

【Differentiation】

Retention of food and stagnation of qi: Epigastric and abdominal distension, hiccups, sticky yellowish coated tongue, rolling forceful pulse. There may be distending pain in the chest and hypochondrium, irritability and wiry forceful pulse.

Attack by pathogenic cold: Slow and forceful hiccup which may be alleviated by hot drinks, white moist tongue coating, slow pulse.

【Treatment】

Prescription: Zusanli, Zhongwan, Neiguan, Geshu, Tiantu.

Points for different syndromes:

Retention of food and stagnation of qi: Neiting, Taihong.

Attack by pathogenic cold: Shangwan (Application of moxibustion).

吃　逆

【弁症】

　実症：多くは食積気滞からなり、上腹部が膨満し、吃逆の音が大きい。舌苔は黄膩で、脈は滑実あるいは弦有力である。

　虚寒症：吃逆の音は緩く有力で、温めると楽になる。舌苔は白く潤い、脈は遅緩である。

【治療】

　処方：足三里、中脘、内関、膈俞、天突。

　症状による配穴：食積気滞によるものは、内庭、太衝。虚寒のものは、上脘に針と灸を併用する。

呕　吐

【辨证】

　饮食停滞：脘腹胀满或疼痛，呕吐酸腐，嗳气厌食，便秘矢气，苔黄厚腻，脉滑实。

　肝气犯胃：呕吐吞酸，嗳气频繁，胸胁胀痛，苔薄腻，脉弦。

　脾胃虚弱：面色萎黄，饮食稍多即吐，食不甘味，大便微溏，神疲肢软，苔薄腻，脉无力。

【治疗】

　处方：足三里、中脘、内关。

　随证配穴：饮食停滞：天枢。
　　　　　　肝气犯胃：太冲。

脾胃虚弱：脾俞。
呕吐不止：金津、玉液（点刺出血，为止呕的经验穴）。

Vomiting

〖Differentiation〗

Retention of food: Epigastric and abdominal distension or pain, acid fermented vomitus, belching, anorexia, constipation, foul gas. The tongue is thickly coated and sticky; the pulse is rolling and forceful.

Invasion of stomach by qi of liver: Vomiting, acid regurgitation, frequent belching, distending pain in hypochondriac region. The tongue is thinly coated and sticky, the pulse wiry.

Weakness of spleen and stomach: Sallow complexion, vomiting after eating a very full meal, lack of appetite, slightly loose stool, general lassitude, forceless pulse, thinly coated, sticky tongue.

〖Treatment〗

Prescription: Zusanli, Zhongwan, Neiguan.
Secondary points:
Retention of food: Tianshu.
Invasion of stomach by qi of liver: Taichong.
Weakness of spleen and stomach: Pishu.
Pernicious vomiting: Jinjin, Yuye.
(Pricking Jinjin, Yuye to cause bleeding is an empirical method for checking vomiting.)

嘔　吐

【弁症】

　飲食停滞：上腹部膨満感あるいは疼痛があり、饐えて腐敗した食物を嘔吐し、噯気があって食欲不振となる。便秘で排気が多い。舌苔は黄色厚膩で、脈は滑実である。
　肝気犯胃：嘔吐、吞酸、噯気が頻繁に発生し、側胸部脹痛。舌苔は薄膩で、脈は弦である。
　脾胃虚弱：顔色が萎黄で、ちょっと食べすぎるとすぐ吐き出す。食事も美味くなく、大便は水様便のようになり、精神が疲れ、四肢無力。舌苔は薄膩で、脈は無力である。

【治療】

　処方：足三里、中脘、内関。
　症状による配穴：飲食停滞：天枢。
　　　　　　　　　肝気犯胃：太衝。
　　　　　　　　　脾胃虚弱：脾俞。
　　　　　　　　　嘔吐不止：金津、玉液。
（点刺して出血させる。止嘔の経験穴である）。

泄　瀉

【辨証】

　急性泄瀉：
　寒湿：大便清稀，腹痛肠鸣，身寒喜温，口不渴，舌淡苔白，脉沉迟。

湿热：大便黄糜热臭，腹痛即泻，肛门灼热，小便短赤，苔黄腻，脉滑数，或兼身热，口渴等。

慢性泄泻：

脾虚：大便溏薄，甚至完谷不化，脘腹胀满，不思饮食，神疲倦怠，苔淡薄，脉细无力。

肾虚：每在黎明前腹微痛，肠鸣泄泻1次或数次，腹及下肢畏寒，苔淡白，脉沉无力。

【治疗】

处方：天枢、足三里、大肠俞。

随证配穴：寒湿：中脘、气海。

湿热：内庭、阴陵泉、合谷。

脾虚：脾俞、中脘。

肾虚：肾俞、太溪、关元、百会、命门。

Diarrhea

【Differentiation】

Acute diarrhea

Cold-damp: Watery diarrhea with abdominal pain and borborygmus, chilliness which responds to warmth, absence of thirst, pale tongue with white coating, deep and slow pulse.

Damp-heat: Diarrhea with yellow, hot, loose and fetid stools, accompanied with abdominal pain, burning sensation in the anus, scanty brownish urine, yellow sticky coated tongue, rolling and rapid pulse. There may be fever and thirst.

Chronic diarrhea

Xu (insufficiency) of yang of spleen: Loose stools with undigested food, epigastric and abdominal distension, anorexia, lassitude, thin white coated tongue, thready forceless pulse.

Xu(insufficiency)of yang of kidney: Slight abdomial pain, borborygmus and diarrhea once or several times each morning at dawn, chilliness in the abdomen and lower extremities, white coated tongue, deep forceless pulse.

【Treatment】

Prescription: Tianshu, Zusanli, Dachangshu
Points for different syndromes:
Cold-damp: Zhongwan, Qihai.
Damp-heat: Neiting, Yinlingquan, Hegu.
Xu of yang of spleen: Pishu, Zhongwan.
Xu of yang of kidney: Shenshu, Taixi, Guanyuan, Baihui, Mingmen.

下　痢

【弁症】

急性下痢:
　寒湿: 大便清稀、腹痛、腸鳴、身体が冷えて、熱いものを好み、口渇がない。舌質は淡く舌苔は白い。脈は沈遅である。
　湿熱: 黄色の熱い穢臭物を排出し、腹が痛んだらすぐ下痢する。肛門に灼熱感あって、小便は短く濃い。舌苔は黄膩。脈は滑数である。あるいは熱と口渇などの症状がある。
　慢性下痢:

脾虚：大便は稀薄で流動状をなし、甚しい時は未消化の食物を排出する。上腹部に膨満感があって、食欲がない。精神的に疲れ、舌苔は淡薄で、脈は細無力である。

腎虚：毎日夜明け前に腹がきりきり痛く、腸がごろごろ鳴り下痢する。回数は1日1回あるいは数回あり、腹部及び下肢に冷感がある。舌苔は淡白。脈は沈無力である。

【治療】

処方：天枢、足三里、大腸俞。
症状による配穴：
　　寒湿：中脘、気海。
　　湿熱：内庭、陰陵泉、合谷。
　　脾虚：脾俞、中脘。
　　腎虚：腎俞、太谿、関元、百会、命門。

便　　秘

【辨证】

实秘：便次减少，三五日间1次，坚涩难下。热结则身热、烦渴、口臭、喜凉，脉滑实。气滞则伴胁腹胀满或疼痛，善叹息，脉弦。

虚秘：属气血虚弱者，伴面唇皖白，神疲，苔薄，脉虚细等。虚寒者伴腹中冷痛，喜热畏寒，脉沉迟。

【治疗】

处方：天枢、支沟、大肠俞、上巨虚。
随证配穴：热结：合谷、曲池。
　　　　　气滞：行间、中脘。

气血虚弱：脾俞、胃俞。
寒秘：气海、关元。

Constipation

【Differentiation】

Shi type: Stool frequency decreases to only once in 3~5 days and difficult to pass. When heat stagnates, the patient may feel hot, thirst, halitosis, preference for cold. The pulse is rolling and forceful. Stagnation of qi is accompanied by distension or pain in the hypochondria and abdomen and sighing, wiry pulse.

Xu type: The patient has a deficiency of both qi and blood, accompanied by pallor of the face and lips, mental fatigue, a thin coated tongue, faintness and a slow pulse. The patient has a feeling of coldness due to Xu(deficiency), accompanied by cold and pain in the abdomen, with a preference for heat over cool conditions. The pulse is deep and slow.

【Treatment】

Prescription: Tianshu, Zhigou, Dachangshu, Shangjuxu.
Points according to symptoms:
Stasis of heat: Hegu, Quchi.
Stagnation of qi: Xingjian, Zhongwan.
Deficiency of both qi and blood: Pishu, Weishu.
Han(cold)type: Qihai, Guanyuan.

便　　秘

【弁症】

実秘：大便の回数が減り、3～5日間に1回、大便が堅まって排便しにくい。熱結あれば発熱し、煩渇があり、口臭があって、冷えるものを好む。脈は滑実である。気滞の場合は、側胸腹部が膨満して、嘆息をよくする。脈は弦である

虚秘：気血の虚弱によるものは、顔と口唇の色がうす白い。精神的に疲れ、舌苔がうすく、脈は虚細である。虚寒のものは、腹の中が冷えて痛み、熱いものを好んで、冷えたものをきらう。脈は沈遅である。

【治療】

処方：天枢、支溝、大腸俞、上巨虚。
症状による配穴：熱結：合谷、曲池。
　　　　　　　　気滞：行間、中脘。
　　　　　　　　気血虚弱：脾俞、胃俞
　　　　　　　　寒秘：気海、関元。

痢　　疾

【辨証】

湿熱痢：腹痛，里急后重，大便染有红白粘冻，或兼有高热，恶心，呕吐。苔黄腻，脉滑数。

寒湿痢：下痢不爽，以白腻粘冻为主，喜暖畏寒，兼有胸脘痞闷，腹中隐痛，口淡不渴，苔白腻，脉沉迟。

久痢：日久不愈，或反复发作，除一般见症外，多兼有精神

疲乏，面色萎黄，怕冷，食欲不振，脉沉细。

【治疗】

处方：天枢、上巨虚、合谷。
随证配穴：湿热：曲池、内庭、阴陵泉。
　　　　　寒湿：中脘、气海、三阴交。
　　　　　久痢：脾俞、胃俞、中脘、足三里。
　　　　　脱肛：百会。

Dysentery

【Differentiation】

Damp-heat type: Abdominal pain, tenesmus, white and red mucus in stool. There may be accompanying symptoms of high fever, nausea and vomiting. Tongue is mostly yellow and sticky coated, pulse rolling and rapid.

Cold-damp type: Scanty defecation, mainly white mucus in stool, response to warmth and dislike of cold, usually with accompanying symptoms of fullness in the chest and epigastrium, lingering abdominal pain, tastelessness in mouth, absence of thirst, white sticky coated tongue, deep slow pulse.

Chronic dysentery: Prolonged persistent dysentery or recurrent dysentery. In addition to the common clinical features, there may be lassitude, sallow complexion, chilliness, anorexia, and deep thready pulse.

【Treatment】

Prescription：Tianshu, Shangjuxu, Hegu.
Points for different syndromes and symptoms：
Damp-heat type：Quchi, Neiting, Yinlingquan.
Cold-damp type：Zhongwan, Qihai, Sanyinjiao.
Chronic dysentery：Pishu, Weishu, Zhongwan, Zusanli.
Prolapse of rectum：Baihui.

細菌性下痢

【弁症】

　湿熱下痢：裏急後重があり、大便に赤と白い粘液がまざっている。あるいは高熱、悪心嘔吐を伴う。舌苔は黄膩で、脈は滑数である。

　寒湿下痢：便意はあるが排便しにくい。大便は白くねばって煮こごりのようなものを主とする。暖いのを好んで、寒いのをおそれ、胸部と上腹部が膨満し、腹がきりきり痛み、口がうすく口渇がない。舌苔は白膩で、脈は沈遅である。

　久痢：下痢が長期間治らず、くり返し発作する。一般の症状のほか、精神的に疲れ、顔色萎黄で、冷えるのをおそれ、食欲不振なども見られる。脈は沈細である。

【治療】

　処方：天枢、上巨虚、合谷。
　症状による配穴：
　　　湿熱：曲池、内庭、陰陵泉。
　　　寒湿：中脘、気海、三陰交。

久痢：脾俞、胃俞、中脘、足三里。
脱肛：百会。

胃 脘 痛

【辨证】

饮食积滞：胃脘胀痛，拒按，嗳气有腐臭味，不思饮食，食则痛甚，苔厚腻，脉沉迟。

肝气犯胃：胃脘阵痛，两胁胀痛，或伴有恶心，呕吐酸水，腹胀，食欲减退，脉沉弦。

胃虚受寒：胃脘隐痛，四肢倦怠，泛吐清水，喜按喜暖，得热则减，舌苔薄白，脉沉迟。

【治疗】

处方：足三里、中脘、内关。
随证配穴：饮食积滞：内庭。
肝气犯胃：太冲。
胃虚受寒：气海（隔姜灸）、脾俞。

Epigastric Pain

【Differentiation】

Retention of food: Distension and pain in the epigastrium, pain aggravated on pressure and after eating, belching with fetid odour, anorexia, thick sticky coated tongue, deep forceful pulse.

Attack on stomach by liver qi: Paroxysmal pain in the epigastrium, distending pain in the hypochondriac region. There may be nausea, acidity, abdominal distension and anorexia. The pulse is deep and wiry.

Xu of stomach with stagnation of cold: Dull pain in the epigastrium, general lassitude, regurgitation of thin fluid, pain which may be alleviated by pressure and warmth, thin white coated tongue, deep slow pulse.

【Treatment】

Prescription: Zusanli, Zhongwan, Neiguan.
Points for different syndromes:
Retention of food: Neiting.
Attack on stomach by liver qi: Taichong.
Xu of stomach with stagnation of cold:
Qihai (indirect moxibustion with ginger) Pishu.

胃脘痛

【弁症】

　飲食が積り滞るもの：上腹部に疼痛があって膨満し、按えられることを拒む。噯気があり、腐敗したようなくさいにおいがする。食欲がなく、飲食すると痛みが激しくなる。舌苔は厚膩。脈は沈実である。

　肝気が胃をおかすもの：上腹部に間歇的な痛みがあり、両側の季肋部に脹痛感があり、あるいは噁心、酸っぱい液を吐き、腹脹、食欲減退などを伴う。脈は沈弦である。

　胃が虚で寒を受けたもの：上腹部にきりきり痛みがあり、四肢倦怠、水液を嘔吐し、按えられると気持がよくなる。熱いも

のを好み、温めると痛みが軽減する。舌苔は薄白。脈は沈遅である。

【治療】

処方：足三里、中脘、内関。
症状による配穴：
　　飲食積滞：内庭。
　　肝気犯胃：太衝。
　　胃虚受寒：気海（生姜隔灸を施す）、脾俞。

黄　　疸

【辨证】

本证以目黄、皮肤黄、小便黄为特征。黄色鲜明的为阳黄，晦暗的为阴黄。阳黄多兼见发热，身重，口渴，腹满，舌苔黄腻，脉象弦数。阴黄多兼见身重，倦怠，嗜睡，口不渴，苔白厚，脉象沉迟。

【治疗】

处方：阴陵泉、足三里、胆俞。
随证配穴：
　　阳黄：太冲、阳陵泉。
　　阴黄：脾俞、三阴交。

Jaundice

【Differentiation】

Jaundice is characterized by yellow sclera, skin

and urine, bright yellow indicating yang type while dark yellow indicates yin type.

Jaundice of yang type is usually accompanied with fever, a heavy sensation of the body, thirst, fullness in the abdomen, yellow sticky coated tongue and wiry rapid pulse.

Jaundice of yin type is usually accompanied by heavy sensation of the body, lassitude, somnolence, absence of thirst, thick white coated tongue and deep slow pulse.

【Treatment】

Prescription: Yinlingquan, Zusanli, Danshu.
Points for different types:
Yang type: Taichong, Yanglingquan.
Yin type: Pishu, Sanyinjiao.

黄　　疸

【弁症】

　本病は、目、皮膚、小便などが黄色くなるのを特徴とする。鮮かな黄色を陽黄とし、晦暗な黄色を陰黄とする。陽黄では、発熱、身重感、口渇、腹部膨満。舌苔が黄膩。脈が弦数などの症状を呈する。陰黄では、身重感、倦怠無力、嗜眠などを兼ね、口渇がない。舌苔は白厚。脈は沈遅である。

【治療】

　処方：陰陵泉、足三里、胆俞。
　症状による配穴：

陽黃：太衝、陽陵泉。
陰黃：脾俞、三陰交。

水　肿

【辨证】

实证：多属急性。一般先肿头面或下肢，皮肤带有光泽，兼有咳喘，发热，口渴，小便短少，腰痛，脉浮或滑数。

虚证：发病较缓，由足跗先肿，也有眼睑先肿，然后遍于全身，兼有怕冷，面色㿠白，腰脊酸痛，四肢无力，腹胀，大便溏薄，脉沉细。

【治疗】

处方：

实证：列缺、合谷、阴陵泉。

虚证：脾俞、肾俞、气海、三阴交、足三里。

随证配穴：面部浮肿：人中。

便秘腹胀：丰隆。

Edema

【Differentiation】

Shi (Excess) type: Onset is usually abrupt. Generally edema appears first on the head, face or lower extremities. The skin is lustrous. Accompanying symptoms and signs are cough, asthma, fever, thirst, scanty urine and low back pain. The pulse is superficial or rolling and rapid.

Xu (Insufficiency) type: Onset is insidious. Edema first appears on the pedis dorsum or eyelids then over the entire body. Accompanying symptoms and signs are chilliness, pallor, backache, general weakness, abdominal distension, loose stools and deep thready pulse.

【Treatment】

Prescription:
Shi type: Lieque, Hegu, Yinlingquan.
Xu type: Pishu, Shenshu, Qihai, Sanyinjiao, Zusanli.
Points according to symptoms:
Edema of the face: Renzhong.
Constipation with abdominal distension: Fenglong.

水　腫

【弁症】

　実症：多くは急性に属ずる。普通はまず頭部、顔面部、あるいは下肢から腫れてくる。皮膚につやがあり、咳、喘息、発熱、口渇などを伴う。小便は短く量が少ない。腰痛がある。脈は浮或は滑数である。

　虚症：発病が比較的に緩慢で、まず足の甲、眼瞼から腫れてくる。次第に全身に及ぶ。冷えるのをおそれ、顔色は白く、腰脊がだるくて痛む。四肢無力、腹部膨満、大便はうすく流動状をなす。脈は沈細である。

【治療】

処方：
　実症：列缺、合谷、陰陵泉。
　虚症：脾俞、腎俞、気海、三陰交、足三里。
症状による配穴：
　顔面部の水腫：人中。
　便秘、腹部膨満：豊隆。

淋　　证

【辨证】

淋证是指小便频数，淋沥刺痛，溲之不尽等言。有兼尿中见血，或尿中夹砂石，或小便浑浊，粘稠如膏；亦有劳累后即发作者。

【治疗】

处方：膀胱俞、中极、阴陵泉、行间、太溪。
随证配穴：尿中见血：血海、三阴交。
　　　　　尿中夹石：委阳、然谷。
　　　　　尿浊如膏：肾俞、照海。
　　　　　劳累即发作：灸百会、气海，去行间。

Stranguria

【Differentiation】

The disease includes frequency of micturition, dribbling, stabbing pain, and incontinence of urine and so on. There are accompanying symptoms of hematuria, or urine containing gravel, or turbid milky urine; exacerbation of symptoms occurs after overworking.

【Treatment】

Prescription: Pangguangshu, Zhongji, Yinglingquan, Xingjian, Taixi.

Points according to symptoms:

Hematuria on urination: Xuehai, Sanyinjiao.

Urine containing gravel: Weiyang, Rangu.

Turbid milky urine: Shenshu, Zhaohai.

Exacerbation of symptoms after overworking: Moxibustion for points of Baihui, Qihai and without Xingjian.

淋　　症

【弁症】

淋症は小便が頻繁で、淋瀝して尿道に刺すような痛みがあり、出渋って断えないなどを指す。尿の中に血が見られ、あるいは砂石もまざり、小便が混濁して、粘稠で脂膏のようになる。疲労するとすぐ起るものもある。

【治療】

処方：膀胱俞、中極、陰陵泉、行間、太谿。
症状による配穴：
　　尿の中に血がまざるもの：血海、三陰交。
　　尿に砂石がまざるもの：委陽、然谷。

尿の混濁したもの：腎俞、照海。
疲労するとすぐ起るもの：百会と気海に灸を施す。

癃　閉

【辨证】

膀胱积热：小便热，量少或尿闭，小腹胀满，口渴不欲饮，或大便不畅，舌红，苔黄，脉数或细数。

经气受损：小便滴沥不畅，或阻塞不通，小腹极度胀满作痛，脉细数，舌有瘀点。

肾阳不足：小便滴沥不爽，排出无力，面色㿠白，神气怯弱，腰膝冷而乏力，舌质淡，脉细弱。

【治疗】

处方：人中、中极、三阴交、外关。
随证配穴：膀胱湿热：阴陵泉。
　　　　　经气受损：血海。
　　　　　肾阳不足：百会、关元。

Retention of Urine

【Differentiation】

Accumulation of damp-heat in the urinary bladder: Hot scanty urine or retention of urine, distension of lower abdomen, thirst but with no desire to drink. Constipation may exist. The tongue is red with yellow coating on the posterior part, the pulse is rapid or thready and rapid.

Damage of the qi of the channels: Dribbling urination or complete retention of urine, distension and pain in the lower abdomen, thready rapid pulse, petechiae over the tongue.

Insufficiency of the yang of the kidney: Dribbling urination with difficulty, pallor, listlessness, chilliness and weakness in the lumbar region and knee, palel tongue, thready pulse especially weak at the proximal part.

【Treatment】

Prescription: Renzhong, Zhongji, Sanyinjiao, Waiguan-Points for different types: Accumulation of damp heat in the urinary bladder: Yinlingquan.
Damage of the qi of the channel: Xuehai.
Insufficiency of the yang of the kidney: Baihui, Guanyuan.

癃　閉

【弁症】

膀胱に湿熱が阻滞されたもの：小便の時に熱感があり、尿の量が少なくなるか尿閉になる。下腹部が膨満し、口渇があっても飲みたくない。あるいは大便不順を伴う。舌質が赤く、舌苔は黄色。脈は数あるいは細数である。

経絡の気が損なわれたもの：小便がしたたり落ちるようで順調でない、あるいは尿路が塞がって通らなくなる。下腹部が極めて膨満して痛い。脈は細数。舌体に瘀血斑点がみられる。

腎陽不足のもの：小便がしたたり落ちるようで排出しにくい。排出無力。顔色は蒼白、精神的に気が弱い。腰膝が冷えて無力。舌質が淡く、脈は細弱である。

【治療】

处方：人中、中極、三陰交、外関。
症状による配穴：
  膀胱湿熱：陰陵泉。
  経気受損：血海。
  腎陽不足：百会、関元。

遺　　尿

【辨证】

夜间在梦中不自觉的排尿，或在遗尿后立即惊醒，有1夜数次，或数夜1次的。一般日久不愈，面色萎黄，食欲不振，肢体乏力等。

【治疗】

处方：膀胱俞、中极、三阴交。
随证配穴：有梦遗尿：神门。
    食欲不振：脾俞、足三里。

Nocturnal Enuresis

【Differentiation】

This is involuntary urination during sleep with

dreams several times a night or once in several nights.
In protracted cases, there are accompanying symptoms
of sallow complexion, anorexia and lassitude.

【Treatment】

Prescription: Pangguangshu, Zhongji, Sanyinjiao.
Points for different symptoms:
Enuresis with dreams: Shenmen.
Anorexia: Pishu, Zusanli.

遺 尿

【弁症】

夜間夢を見ている間に尿が無意識に排出され、あるいは遺尿した後すぐに目がさめる。1夜に数回または数夜に1回遺尿をする。もし長期間治らなければ、顔色萎黄、食欲不振、肢体脱力感などの症状がある。

【治療】

処方：膀胱俞、中極、三陰交。
症状による配穴：
　　夢中遺尿：神門。
　　食欲不振：脾俞、足三里。

阳 痿

【辨证】

阳痿是以阴茎萎弱不能勃起为主证。肾阳不足，多见面色㿠

白，头晕目眩，精神不振，腰腿酸软，小便频数，脉多沉细；如兼心脾虚者，则有心悸胆怯，失眠等。

【治疗】

处方：关元、中极、太溪、百会、肾俞。
随证配穴：心脾虚：心俞、神门、三阴交。

Impotence

【Differentiation】

Impotence is characterized by inability of the penis to erect. In case of insufficiency of yang of kidney. Pallor, dizziness, blurring of vision, listlessness soreness and weakness of the lumbar region and knee frequent urination and deep thready pulse may appear. If it is complicated with damage of qi of the heart and spleen, palpitation and insomnia may be present.

【Treatment】

Prescription: Guanyuan, Zhongji, Taixi, Baihui, Shenshu.

Points for damage of qi of heart and spleen: Xinshu, Shenmen, Sanyinjiao.

陰萎

【弁症】

陰萎は陰茎が萎え、勃起不能を主症とする。腎陽不足の場合には、顔色皓白、眩暈、精神不振、腰と下肢がだるくて力が

ない。頻尿、脈が沈細などがよく見られ、心脾の損傷を兼ねるものには、心悸、びくびくし、不眠などの症がある。

【治療】

処方：関元、中極、太谿、百会、腎俞。
症狀による配穴：
　　心脾虛：心俞、神門、三陰交。

遺　　精

【辨证】

梦遗：多梦有所感而遗精，每于遗精后，次日头晕，心悸，精神不振，体倦乏力，小便黄短，舌红，脉细数。
滑精：滑精频作，面色㿠白，精神萎靡，舌淡，脉沉弱无力。

【治疗】

处方：关元、神門、三阴交。
随证配穴：梦遗：内关。
　　　　　滑精：肾俞、足三里。

Seminal Emission

【Differentiation】

Nocturnal emission: Seminal emission may be with dreams."Morning-after"dizziness,palpitation,listlessness, lassitude, scanty yellow urine, red tongue and thready rapid pulse.

Involuntary emission: Frequent emission, pallor, listlessness,pale tongue,deep feeble forceless pulse.

【Treatment】

Prescription: Guanyuan, Shenmen, Sanyinjiao.
Points for different types:
Nocturnal emission: Neiguan.
Involuntary emission: Shenshu, Zusanli.

遺　　精

【弁症】

　夢精：多くは夢を見ている時、多少自覚があって遺精し、遺精した次の日は眩暈、心悸、精神不振、倦怠無力、小便が短く色は黄色などを現わし、舌質が赤く、脈は細数である。

　滑精：夢を伴わない遺精である。頻繁に遺精し、顔色蒼白、精神的におちこむなどの症状がある。舌質はうすく、脈は沈弱無力である。

【治療】

　処方：関元、神門、三陰交。
　症状による配穴：
　　夢精：内関。
　　滑精：腎俞、足三里。

中　　风

【辨证】

　在脏腑：属于中风的重证，可分闭证与脱证。

— 189 —

闭证：突然跌倒，昏迷不省，眼开，两手握紧，牙关紧闭，面热，耳赤，痰多，呼吸气粗，大便秘结，小便不通，脉弦滑有力。

脱证：跌倒昏迷，两手撒开，口开，眼合，面色苍白，头面出汗，甚则大小便失禁，四肢厥冷，脉虚。

在经络：属于中风的轻证，一般仅为部分肢体运动不利，或一部分肌肤知觉减退，见半身不遂或口㖞等症。

【治疗】

处方：

闭证：人中、百会、涌泉、手十二井穴。

随证配穴：牙关紧闭：颊车、下关、合谷。

痰多：天突、丰隆。

舌强不语：哑门、廉泉、通里。

脱证：气海、关元、人中、足三里。

随证配穴：半身不遂：百会、风府。

上肢：肩髃、曲池、外关、合谷。

下肢：环跳、阳陵泉、足三里、解溪。

口眼㖞斜：参见"口眼㖞斜"证。

Windstroke

【Differentiation】

The severe type, the zang-fu organs being attacked, may be subdivided into tense syndrome and flaccid syndrome.

Tense syndrome: Sudden collapse, coma, staring eyes, clenched fists and jaws, redness of face and ears, gurgling with sputum, coarse breathing, retention of urine, constipation, wiry and rolling forceful pulse.

Flaccid syndrome: Coma, hands relaxed and mouth agape, eyes closed, pallor, sweat over head and face. There may be incontinence of feces and urine, cold limbs and feeble pulse.

The mild type, channels and collaterals being attacked. Manifestations are hemiplegia or deviation of mouth due to motor or sensory impairment.

【Treatment】

Prescription:
Tense syndrome: Renzhong, Baihui, Yongquan, the 12 Jing-Well Points of both hands.
Points according to symptoms and signs:
Clenched jaws: Jiache, Xiaguan, Hegu.
Gurgling with sputum: Tiantu, Fenglong.
Aphasia and stiffness of tongue: Yamen, Lianquan, Tongli.
Flaccid syndrome: Qihai, Guanyuan, Renzhong, Zusanli.
Hemiplegia: Baihui, Fengfu.
Upper extremity: Jianyu, Quchi, Waiguan, Hegu.
Lower extremity: Huantiao, Yanglingquan, Zusanli, Jiexi.
Facial paralysis: (See the following treatment of Facial Paralysis.)

卒 中

【弁症】

臓腑にある：ひどい卒中に属する。閉症と脱症の2種類に分けられる。

閉症：急に卒倒、昏迷し、目をあけ、両手は拳を握り、歯をくいしばる。顔面に熱感があり、耳も赤くなる。痰が多く、呼吸も荒くなり、大便秘結し、小便も不通になる。脈は弦滑で力が強い。

脱症：卒倒、昏迷し、両手をだらりと開き、口は開き、目を閉じ、顔色蒼白で、頭部と顔面部にあぶら汗が出る。甚しきは大小便ともに失禁し、四肢がつめたく、脈は虚である。

経絡にある：軽い卒中に属する。普通は一部の肢体運動が不自由になり、またはある部分の皮膚が無感覚になる。そのため、半身不遂、あるいは口が歪むなどの症状が現われる。

【治療】

処方：
閉症：人中、百会、湧泉、手十二井穴。
症状による配穴：
    歯をくいしばる場合：頬車、下関、合谷。
    痰が多い場合：天突、豊隆。
    言語障碍の場合：瘂門、廉泉、通里。
脱症：気海、関元、人中、足三里。
症状に応る配穴：
    半身不遂：百会、風府。
    上肢：肩髃、曲池、外関、合谷。
    下肢：環跳、陽陵泉、足三里、解谿。

口眼歪斜：口眼歪斜の項参照。

口 眼 歪 斜

【辨证】

病侧眼睑闭合不全，流泪，口角下垂，流涎，不能皱额，蹙眉，闭眼，鼓腮，示齿和吹哨等；部分病人有耳根后疼痛或头痛。苔薄白，脉浮。

【治疗】

处方：翳风、地仓、颊车、阳白、太阳、合谷、颧髎、下关。

随证配穴：头痛：风池。
皱额皱眉差：攒竹、丝竹空。
闭目不全：睛明、瞳子髎、鱼腰。
耸鼻不能：迎香。
人中沟歪斜：人中。
耳鸣耳聋：听会。
口眼瞤动：太冲。

Facial Paralysis

【Differentiation】

Clinical manifestations on the affected side are incomplete closing of the eye, lacrimation, dropping of the angle of the mouth, salivation, and inability to frown, raise the eyebrow close the eye, blow out the cheek, show the teeth or whistle. There may be pain in the mastoid region or headache. The tongue is coated white. The pulse is superficial.

【Treatment】

Prescription: Yifeng, Dicang, Jiache, Yangbai Taiyang, Hegu Quanliao, Xiaguan.

Points according to symptoms and signs:
Headache: Fengchi.
Difficulty in frowning and raising the eyebrow: Zanzhu, Sizhukong.
Incomplete closing of the eye: Jingming, Tongziliao, Yuyao.
Difficulty in sniffling: Yingxiang.
Deviation of the philtrum: Renzhong.
Tinnitus and deafness: Tinghui.
Twitching of the eyelid and the mouth: Taichong.

口眼歪邪

【弁症】

患側の目をしっかり閉じることができなくなり、流涙、口角下垂、流涎、しわを寄せることとまゆをひそめることが出来なくなり、ふくれっつら様の感じになり、歯を露出し、口笛を吹くことなどもできなくなる。病人によっては耳の後に痛みがあり、頭痛の症狀もある。舌苔は薄白。脈は浮である。

【治療】

処方：翳風、地倉、頬車、陽白、太陽、合谷、顴髎、下関。

症状による配穴：

頭痛：風池。

しわを寄せるとまゆをひそめることなどができないもの：攢竹、絲竹空。

目をしっかり閉じることができないもの：睛明、瞳子髎、魚腰。

鼻翼を動かすことができないもの：迎香。

人中溝がずれている場合：人中。

耳鳴、難聴：聴会。

口と目がぴくぴく動いている場合：太衝。

头　　痛

【辨证】

根据头痛部位，辨别病患所在的经络。如头痛主要在后头部及颈部的，与太阳经有关；主要在前额，眉棱骨部的，与阳明经有关；在两额角或偏一侧的，与少阳经有关；在巅顶部，与厥阴经有关。

【治疗】

用局部与远道循经配穴法，以祛风，通络，调和气血。

处方：后头痛：风池、昆仑、后溪。

前头痛：头维、印堂、上星、合谷、内庭。

偏头痛：太阳、率谷、外关、足临泣。

— 195 —

头顶痛：百会、后溪、至阴、太冲。
随证配穴：肝阳上亢：行间、阳陵泉。
气血虚弱：气海、足三里。

Headache

【Differentiation】

Headache is differentiated according to its locality and its supplying channels. Pain at the occipital region and neck, for example, is related to Urinary Bladder Channel of Foot-Taiyang, pain at the forehead and supraorbital region relates to the Stomach Channel of Foot-Yangming, pain at the temporal region of both sides or only one side relates to the Gall bladder Channel of Foot-Shaoyang and that at the parietal region is related to the Liver Channel of Foot-Jueyin.

【Treatment】

To dispel wind, remove obstruction in the channels and collaterals, and regulate qi and blood by puncturing points of the local area combined with points of the remote area.

Prescription:

Occipital headache: Fengchi, Kunlun, Houxi.

Frontal headache: Touwei, Yintang, Shangxing, Hegu, Neiting.

One-side headache: Taiyang, Shuaigu, Waiguan, Foot-Linqi.

Parietal headache: Baihui, Houxi, Zhiyin, Taichong.

Points according to symptoms and signs:
Hyperactivity of yang of liver:Xingjian, Yanglingquan.
Deficiency of qi and blood:Qihai, Zusanli.

頭　　痛

【弁症】

頭痛の部位によって、疾患の所在する経絡を弁別する。すなわち頭痛が後頭部、頸部にある場合は、太陽経と関連があり、前頭部にある場合は、陽明経、両側或は片方にある場合は、少陽経、頭頂部にある場合は、厥陰経と関連がある。

【治療】

経絡に沿って局部と遠隔の経穴をくみあわせて取り、風を取り除き、経絡を通らせ、気血を調和する。
処方：後頭痛：風池、崑崙、後谿。
　　　前頭痛：頭維、印堂、上星、合谷、内庭。
　　　偏頭痛：太陽、率谷、外関、足臨泣。
　　　頭頂痛：百会、後谿、至陰、太衝。
症状による配穴：
　　　肝陽上亢：行間、陽陵泉。
　　　気血虚弱：気海、足三里。

眩　　暈

【辨証】

主要症状为头晕，眼花，伴有自身或视物旋转感，站立则欲

— 197 —

倒。

肝阳上亢：多兼见耳鸣，面赤，恶心，腰酸，舌质红，脉弦数。

痰湿内停：兼见胸脘满闷，呕恶痰多，食欲不振，苔白腻，脉滑。

气血两虚：兼见精神不振，四肢无力，心悸，失眠，脉虚而无力。

【治疗】

处方：肝阳上亢：肾俞、太溪、肝俞、行间、风池。
　　　痰湿内停：脾俞、中脘、丰隆、内关、头维。
　　　气血两虚：关元、脾俞、三阴交、足三里。

Dizziness and Vertigo

【Differentiation】

Main Symptoms are giddiness, and blurring of vision with a whirling sensation and of things turning, also of a tendency to fall.

Upward attack of hyperactive yang of liver: Besides the main symptoms, there appear tinnitus, flushed face, nausea, backache, redness of tongue proper and wiry and rapid pulse.

Interior retention of phlegm-damp: Complications are fullness and suffocating sensation of chest and epigastric region, nausea and vomiting, profuse sputum anorexia, white and sticky coated tongue, rolling pulse.

Xu (deficiency) of qi and blood: Complications are listlessness, lassitude, palpitation, insomnia, weak pulse.

【Treatment】

Prescription:

Upward attack of hyperactive yang of liver: Shenshu, Taixi, Ganshu, Xingjian, Fengchi.

Interior retention of phlegm-damp: Pishu, Zhongwan, Fenglong, Neiguan, Touwei.

Xu (deficiency) of qi and blood: Guanyuan, Pishu, Sanyinjiao, Zusanli.

眩　　暈

【弁症】

主な症状は眩暈、目がかすみ、頭がくらくらして、周囲のものが回転するような感じで、立つと倒れそうな症状がある。

肝陽上亢：耳鳴、顔色が赤く。悪心、腰がだるい。舌質は赤く、脈は弦数などの症状が見られる。

痰湿内停：胸が重苦しく。嘔吐、嗯心、痰が多い。食欲も不振。舌苔は白膩。脈は滑などの症状がみられる。

気血両虚：精神不振、四肢無力、心悸、不眠。脈は虚無力などの症状が見られる。

【治療】

処方：肝陽上亢：腎兪、太谿、肝兪、行間、風池。
　　　痰湿内停：脾兪、中脘、豊隆、内関、頭維。
　　　気血両虚：関元、脾兪、三陰交、足三里。

心悸、怔忡

心悸时作时止者,病情较轻;如病情比较重,表现为心胸跳动,不能自主,无休止时,则为怔忡。

【辨证】

气血不足:面色苍白,气短,乏力,夜寐不宁,头晕目眩,舌胖淡有齿痕,脉细无力。
痰火内动:见烦躁不宁,恍惚多梦,苔黄,脉滑数。
水饮内停:咳吐痰涎,胸脘痞满,精神倦怠,苔白,脉弦滑。

【治疗】

处方:心俞、神门、内关。
随证配穴:气血不足:气海、脾俞、胃俞。
　　　　　痰火内动:丰隆、阳陵泉。
　　　　　水饮内停:关元、足三里、膻中。

【参考】

本证可见于神经官能症和植物神经紊乱,以及各种心脏病引起的心律失常。

Palpitation, Anxiety

In mild cases, palpitation may be intermittent; in severe cases, there may be continuous and incontrollable violent throbbing of the heart.

【Differentiation】

Insufficiency of qi and blood: Pallor, shortness of breath, general weakness, disturbed sleep, dizziness, blurring of vision, pale flabby tongue with teeth prints on the border, thready forceless pulse.

Stirring of endogenous phlegm-fire: Irritability, restlessness, dream-disturbed sleep, yellow coated tongue, rolling rapid pulse.

Retention of harmful fluid: Expectoration of mucoid sputum, fullness in the chest and epigastric region, lassitude, white coated tongue, wiry rolling pulse.

【Treatment】

Prescription: Xinshu, Shenmen, Neiguan.
Points according to syndromes:
Insufficiency of qi and blood: Qihai, Pishu, Weishu.
Stirring of endogenous phlegm-fire: Fenglong, Yanglingquan.
Retention of harmful fluid: Guanyuan, Zusanli, Shanzhong.

【Remarks】

Palpitation and anxiety described here may be symptoms present in neurosis, functional disorders of vegetative nervous system and cardiac arrhythmia of various origins.

心悸、怔忡

心悸が発作したり、よくなったりするのは、病状が軽いほ

うて，心悸と称する。もし心臓の搏動が酷くて，押えられなくなり，止められず発作するのは，怔忡と称し，病状のわりに重くなったものである。

【弁症】

気血不足：顔面蒼白、気短、無力、不眠、眩暈。舌体が肥大し、かつ歯痕があり、脈は細無力である。

痰火内動：煩躁不安、頭がぼうっとして夢が多い。舌苔は黄色。脈は滑数である。

水飲内停：咳があって、痰液が多い。上腹部に膨満感があり、精神倦怠などが見られる。舌苔は白く、脈は弦滑である。

【治療】

処方：心俞、神門、内関。
症状による配穴：
　　気血不足：気海、脾俞、胃俞。
　　痰火内動：豊隆、陽陵泉。
　　水飲内停：関元、足三里、膻中。

【参考】

本症はノイローゼ症あるいは自律神経系の機能異常及び各種心臓病により引き起された心搏動異常などに見られる。

癲　狂

【辨证】

癲证发病缓慢，初起先有精神苦闷，神志呆滞，继则言语错乱，哭笑无常，或终日不语，喜静多睡，不思饮食，舌苔薄或厚

腻，脉弦细。

狂证发病较为急速，病前亦见烦躁易怒，少睡少食，继而狂躁好动，高声叫骂，弃衣奔走，终日不眠；甚者毁物打人，苔黄腻，脉弦滑而数。

【治疗】

处方：癫证：神门、内关、心俞、丰隆、太冲。
　　　狂证：人中、内关、合谷、丰隆、太冲。

【参考】

本证可见于精神分裂症。

Depressive and Manic Mental Disorders

【Differentiation】

Depressive mental disorder: Gradual onset, mental depression and dullness at the initial stage, followed by paraphasia and paraphronia, or muteness, hypersomnia and anorexia. The tongue is thinly or moderately coated. The pulse is wiry and thready.

Manic mental disorder: Sudden onset, preceded by irritability, peevishness, scarcely sleeping and eating. This is followed by mania demonstrated by shouting, yelling, tearing off clothes, running about, sleeplessness, smashing things and hitting people. The tongue is yellow and sticky. The pulse is usually wiry, rolling and rapid.

【Treatment】

Prescription:
Depressive mental disorder: Shenmen, Neiguan, Xinshu, Fenglong, Taichong.
Manic mental disorder: Renzhong, Neiguan, Hegu, Fenglong, Taichong.

【Remarks】

Depressive and manic mental disorders correspond to the depressive and manic types of schizophrenia in modern medicine.

癲　狂

【弁症】

癲症は、発病が緩慢で、早期では、精神状態が苦しく、いらいらして、神志がにぶくなり、次第に言語錯乱、泣いたり笑ったり、或は終日無言、静かなことを好み、よく眠り、食欲がないなどの症状が見られる。舌苔は薄く、または厚膩で、脈は弦細である。

狂症は、発病がわりに急速で、発病前はいらいらして怒りやすい。睡眠が少なく飲食も少ない。続いて狂躁して激動しやすくなり、人を口汚く罵り、裸で駆けまわり、終日不眠などの症状が見られる。甚しくなると、物をこわしたり、人を傷付けることもある。舌苔は黄膩で、脈は多く弦滑かつ数である。

【治療】

処方：癲症：神門、内関、心俞、豊隆、太衝。
　　　狂症：人中、内関、合谷、豊隆、太衝。

【参考】

本症は、精神分裂症に見られる。

不　寐

【辨证】

脾虚血少：难于入睡，易惊醒，兼有心悸，健忘，四肢无力，精神不振，食欲减退，面色萎黄，脉细无力。
心肾不交：心烦，失眠，兼有头昏，耳鸣，腰酸，遗精，白带，脉虚数。
肝火上扰：性情急躁抑郁，睡中多梦，兼有头痛，胸胁胀痛，口苦，脉弦。
胃气不和：失眠兼有脘部满闷，腹胀，嗳气，脉实有力。

【治疗】

处方：神门、内关、三阴交。
随证配穴：脾虚血少：脾俞、心俞、隐白。
　　　　　心肾不交：心俞、肾俞、太溪。
　　　　　肝火上扰：肝俞、太冲。
　　　　　胃气不和：胃俞、足三里。

Insomnia

【Differentiation】

Xu of spleen and blood insufficiency: Difficulty in falling asleep and disturbed sleep accompanied by palpitation, poor memory, lassitude, listlessness, anorexia, sallow complexion and thready weak pulse.

Disharmony of heart and kidney: Irritability and insomnia accompanied by dizziness, tinnitus, low back pain, seminal emission, leukorrhagia and rapid weak pulse.

Upward disturbance of liver fire: Mental depression, quick temper and dream-disturbed sleep accompanied by headache, distending pain in the costa and hypochondrium, bitter taste in mouth and wiry pulse.

Dysfunction of stomach: Insomnia accompanied by fullness in the epigastric region and suffocating feeling, abdominal distension, belching and full forceful pulse.

【Treatment】

Prescription: Shenmen, Neiguan, Sanyinjiao.

Points according to different syndromes:

Xu of spleen and blood insufficiency: Pishu, Xinshu Yinbai.

Disharmony of heart and kidney: Xinshu Shenshu, Taixi.

Upward disturbance of liver fire: Ganshu, Taichong.

Dysfunction of stomach: Weishu, Zusanli.

不　眠

【弁症】

脾虚血少：ねつきが悪く、目がさめやすい。また心悸、健忘、四肢無力、精神不振、食欲減退などを兼ねる。顔色は萎黄で、脈は細無力である。

心腎不交：心煩、不眠で、頭昏、耳鳴、腰がだるい。遺精、帯下などがある。脈は虚数である。

肝火上擾：情緒がせっかち或は抑うつで、夢が多く、頭痛、側胸部の膨満と疼痛、口が苦いなどの症状を兼ねる。脈は弦である。

胃気不和：不眠で、上腹部膨満感、腹脹、噯気などの症状を兼ねる。脈は実かつ有力である。

【治療】

処方：神門、内関、三陰交。

症状による配穴：

脾虚血少：脾兪、心兪、隠白。
心腎不交：心兪、腎兪、太谿。
肝火上擾：肝兪、太衝。
胃気不和：胃兪、足三里。

胁　痛

【辨证】

气滞：胁肋胀痛，胸闷不舒，口苦，脉弦，症状往往随情志的变化而增减。

血瘀：胁痛如刺，入夜更甚，痛处不移，并且拒按，舌有紫色斑点，脉弦。

【治疗】

处方：阳陵泉、支沟、期门。
随证配穴：气滞：肝俞、足临泣。
　　　　　血瘀：膈俞、行间。

Hypochondriac Pain

【Differentiation】

Stagnation of qi: Distending pain in the costa and hypochondrium, fullness in the chest, bitter taste in mouth, wiry pulse. Severity of symptoms varies with emotional state.

Stagnation of blood: Fixed stabbing pain in the hypochondrium, pain intensified on pressure and at night, purplish petechiae on the tongue, wiry pulse.

【Treatment】

Prescription: Yanglingquan, Zhigou, Qimen.
Points for different types:
Stagnation of qi: Ganshu, Foot-Linqi.
Stagnation of blood: Geshu, Xingjiang.

脇　　痛

【弁症】

気滞：季肋部が膨満して痛みがあり、胸悶かつ不快感が現われ、口が苦い。脈は弦である。症状は往往情緒の変化により軽減したり、悪くなったりする。

血淤：季肋部に針を刺すような痛みがあり、部位は固定して、夜になると激しくなる。局所は按さえられることを拒む。舌体に紫色の斑点があり、脈は弦である。

【治療】

処方：陽陵泉、支溝、期門。
症状による配穴：
　　気滞：肝俞、足臨泣。
　　血淤：膈俞、行間。

腹　　痛

【辨証】

寒邪内積：痛势急暴，喜暖，便溏，苔白，脉沉紧。
饮食停滞：脘腹胀满，痛处拒按，嗳腐吞酸，或者痛而欲泻，泻后痛减，苔腻，脉滑。

【治疗】

处方：脐上痛：下脘、足三里。
　　　当脐痛：天枢、气海。
　　　少腹痛：关元、三阴交。

【参考】

对由急腹症引起的急重腹痛，应严密观察，并采取其他治疗措施。

Abdominal Pain

【Differentiation】

Internal accumulation of cold: Sudden violent pain which responds to warmth, loose stools, white coated tongue, deep tense pulse.

Retention of food: Epigastric and abdominal distension and pain which may be aggravated by pressure, foul belching and acidity. Abdominal pain may be accompanied by diarrhea and relieved after defecation. The tongue is sticky coated; the pulse is rolling.

【Treatment】

Prescriptions:
Pain above the umbilicus: Xiawan, Zusanli.
Pain around the umbilicus: Tianshu, Qihai.
Pain in the lower abdomen: Guanyuan, Sanyinjiao.

【Remark】

For acute, severe abdominal pain caused by acute abdomen, strict observation of the patient is necessary and other therapeutic measures should be taken when necessary.

腹　　痛

【弁症】

　寒邪内積：急にひどい痛みが出て、熱いのを好む。大便は水様流動状。舌苔が白く、脈は沈緊である。

　飲食停滞：上腹部に膨満感があり、痛む所は、按さえられることを拒み、噯気に腐敗したようなにおいが出る。吞酸、あるいは痛んだら下痢し、下痢した後は痛みが軽減する。舌苔は膩、脈は滑である。

【治療】

　処方：臍の上部の疼痛：下脘、足三里。
　　　　臍部の疼痛：天枢、気海。
　　　　下腹の疼痛：関元、三陰交。

【参考】

　急性腹症により引き起された急重腹痛は、まず厳密に観察すべきで、他の救急手当も考えなければならない。

腰　　痛

【辨证】

　寒湿：多发于感受风寒湿邪之后，腰背重痛，肌肉拘急不能俯仰；或痛连臀部下肢，病部常觉寒冷，每遇阴雨天则加重，卧床休息症状亦不减轻。

　肾虚：病起缓慢，痛势缓和，日久不愈，精神倦怠，腰膝无力，劳倦则症状显著加剧，卧床休息后很快可以缓解。

外伤：有腰部扭伤史，腰脊强痛，一般痛处都固定不移，手按或转侧时则疼痛更甚。

【治疗】

处方：肾俞、腰阳关、委中。
随证配穴：肾虚：命门、太溪。
扭伤腰脊强痛：人中。

Low Back Pain

【Differentiation】

Cold-damp: Low back pain usually occurs after exposure to pathogenic wind, cold and damp. Clinical manifestations are heavy sensation and pain in the dorsolumbar region and stiffness of muscles, limiting extension and flexion of the back. The pain may reflex downward to the buttocks and lower extremities, and the cold sensation over the affected area. Pain becomes intensified in cloudy and rainy days and is not alleviated by bed rest.

Xu (insufficiency) of qi of kidney: Onset is insidious, and pain is mild but protracted, with lassitude and weakness of the lumbar region and knee. Symptoms are intensified after strain and stress and alleviated by bed rest.

Trauma: The patient has a history of sprain of the lumbar region. Clinical manifestations are rigidity and pain of the lower back. The pain is fixed and aggravated on pressure and turning of the body.

【Treatment】

Prescription：Shenshu, Yaoyangguan, Weizhong.
Secondary points：
Xu(insufficiency)of qi of kidney：Mingmen, Taixi.
Sprain of the lumbar region：Renzhong.

腰　　痛

【弁症】

　寒湿：多くは風寒湿邪を感受した後に発病する。腰背が重くて痛みがあり、筋肉痙攣のため、起居動作ができなくなる。或は殿部、下肢まで牽引痛が出て、腰部に冷感があらわれる。雨天には痛みが激しくなり、寝かせて安静にしても症状が軽減しない。

　腎虚：発病が緩慢で、進行も緩和である。長期間に治らないで、精神倦怠感、腰膝無力などを伴う。また疲労の後は更に酷くなり、寝かせて休んだら近いうちに症状が緩和する。

　外傷：腰部が損傷されたことにより、腰椎に激しい疼痛が出る。疼痛部位は一般に固定して移動しない。局所を押えたり、あるいは運動すると痛みは更に激しくなる。

【治療】

　処方：腎俞、腰陽関、委中。
　症状による配穴：
　　　腎虚：命門、太谿。
　　　ギックリ腰の激しい疼痛に：人中。

痹 证

【辨证】

主证是关节酸痛,或一部分肌肉酸痛麻木,日久不愈,可发生肢体拘挛,甚至关节肿大或变形等。

【治疗】

根据病痛部位,局部取穴。

处方：肩关节痛：肩髃，肩髎，肩贞，臑俞。

肘臂痛：曲池、尺泽、外关、合谷。

髋关节部痛：环跳、殷门、居髎。

膝关节痛：梁丘、犊鼻、阳陵泉、阴陵泉。

小腿麻痛：承山、飞扬。

踝部痛：解溪、丘墟、昆仑、太溪。

腰脊痛：腰阳关。

全身痛：后溪、申脉、大包、膈俞。

随证配穴：发热配大椎、骨节变形配大杼。

【参考】

本证可见于风湿热，风湿性关节炎，类风湿性关节炎等。

Bi Syndrome

【Differentiation】

The chief symptom is arthralgia. There may be muscular soreness and numbness. In prolonged cases, contracture of the extremities, or even swelling or deformity of joints may be present.

【Treatment】

Selection of local points should be taken according to the diseased areas.

Prescriptions:

Pain in the shoulder joint: Jianyu, Jianliao, Jianzhen, Naoshu.

Pain in the elbow: Quchi, Chize, Waiguan, Hegu.

Pain in the hip joint: Huantiao, Yinmen, Juliao.

Pain in the knee joint: Liangqiu, Dubi, Yanglingquan, Yinlingquan.

Numbness and pain in the leg: Chengshan, Feiyang.

Pain in the ankle: Jiexi, Qiuxu, Kunlun, Taixi.

Pain in the lumbar region: Yaoyangguan.

General aching: Houxi, Shenmai, Dabao, Geshu.

Points according to symptoms and signs:

Fever: Dazhui.

Deformity of the joint: Dashu.

【Remark】

Bi syndrome may be seen in rheumatic fever, rheumatic arthritis, rheumatoid arthritis.

痺　症

【弁症】

痺症の主症は関節がだるくて痛い。あるいは一部の筋肉がだるくてしびれるのであるが、短期間で治らなければ、肢体が

ひきつり、ひどくなると関節がはれあがり、或は変形する。

【治療】

疼痛の部位により、局部で穴を取る。
処方：
　　　　肩関節痛：肩髃、肩髎、肩貞、臑俞。
　　　　肘臂痛：曲池、尺沢、外関、合谷。
　　　　股関節部痛：環跳、殷門、居髎。
　　　　膝関節痛：梁丘、犢鼻、陽陵泉、陰陵泉。
　　　　小腿のしびれ：承山、飛揚。
　　　　足関節痛：解谿、丘墟、崑崙、太谿。
　　　　腰背痛：腰陽関。
　　　　全身痛：後谿、申脈、大包、膈俞。
症状による配穴：
　　　　発熱：大椎。
　　　　骨が変形する場合：大杼。

【参考】

本症は、リューマチ熱、リューマチ性関節炎、リューマチ様性関節炎などに見られる。

痿　証

【辨証】

四肢筋肉弛緩无力，甚至萎縮，从而失去运动功能为主证。

肺热：多发生在热病中或热病后，兼有咳嗽，心烦，口渴，小便短赤，舌红苔黄，脉细数。

湿热：兼有面黄神疲，小便混浊，或双足发热，得冷则舒，

苔黄腻，脉实。

　　肝肾阴亏：兼有腰膝酸软，遗精早泄，带下，头晕、目眩、舌红、脉细数。

【治疗】

　　处方：上肢：肩髃、曲池、合谷、外关。
　　　　　下肢：髀关、足三里、解溪、环跳、阳陵泉、悬钟。
　　随证配穴：肺热：尺泽、肺俞。
　　　　　　　湿热：脾俞、阴陵泉。
　　　　　　　肝肾不足：肝俞、肾俞。

【参考】

　　本证可见于急性脊髓炎，进行性肌萎缩，重症肌无力，周期性麻痹，癔病性瘫痪等。

Wei Syndrome

【Differentiation】

Wei syndrome is characterized by muscular flaccidity or atrophy of the extremities with motor impairment.

Heat in the lung: It usually occurs during or after a febrile disease, and is accompanied by cough, irritability, thirst, scanty brownish urine, red tongue with yellow coating, and thready rapid pulse.

Damp-heat: The accompanying symptoms and signs are sallow complexion, listlessness and cloudy urine. There may be a hot sensation in the soles of the feet with desire to expose them to coolness. Yellow and sticky coated tongue, forceful pulse.

Insufficiency of the essence of the liver and kidney: The accompanying symptoms are soreness and weakness of the lumbar region, seminal emission, prospermia, leukorrhea, dizziness and blurring of vision, red tongue, thready rapid pulse.

【Treatment】

Prescriptions:
Upper limb: Jianyu, Quchi, Hegu, Waiguan.
Lower limb: Piguan, Zusanli, Jiexi, Huantiao, Yanglingquan, Xuanzhong.
Points for different types:
Heat in the lung: Chize, Feishu.
Damp-heat: Pishu, Yinlingquan.
Insufficiency of essence of liver and kidney: Ganshu, Shenshu.

【Remark】

Wei syndrome is seen in acute myelitis, progressive myatrophy, myasthenia gravis, periodic paralysis and hysterical paralysis.

萎　症

【弁症】

　　四肢の筋肉が弛緩無力で、甚しくなると萎縮し、運動機能を失うようになる。

　　肺熱：熱性病中あるいは熱性病後に発生する。咳嗽、心

煩、口渇などの症状を兼ね、小便は少なく赤い。舌質は赤く、舌苔は黄色で、脈は細数である。

湿熱：顔色が黄色で倦怠感があり、小便は混濁し、足に熱感があって、冷やすと快適になる。舌苔は黄膩で、脈は実である。

肝腎陰虧：腰背がだるく、遺精早漏、白帯下、頭暈、目眩などの症状を兼ねる。舌質が赤く、脈は細数である。

【治療】

処方：上肢：肩髃、曲池、合谷、外関。
　　　下肢：髀関、足三里、解谿、環跳、陽陵泉、懸鐘。
症状による配穴：
　肺熱：尺沢、肺俞。
　湿熱：脾俞、陰陵泉。
　肝腎陰虧：肝俞、腎俞。

【参考】

本症は、急性脊髄炎、進行性筋肉萎縮、重症筋無力症、周期性麻痺、ヒステリー性麻痺などの疾患に見られる。

扭挫伤

【辨证】

局部酸胀疼痛，或轻微红肿，活动受限，重则不能转动。

【治疗】

处方：阿是穴。
随证配方：颈项：天柱、后溪。

肩关节：肩井、肩髃。
　　肘关节：曲池、合谷。
　　腕关节：阳池、外关。
　　股关节：环跳、阳陵泉。
　　膝关节：犊鼻、内庭。
　　踝关节：解溪、丘墟、昆仑。

Sprain

【Differentiation】

Local soreness, distension and pain or mild redness and swelling. Movement is limited or impossible.

【Treatment】

Prescription: Ashi Points.
Secondary points:
Neck: Tianzhu, Houxi.
Shoulder joint: Jianjing, Jianyu.
Elbow joint: Quchi, Hegu.
Wrist joint: Yangchi, Waiguan.
Hip joint: Huantiao, Yanglingquan.
Knee joint: Dubi, Neiting.
Ankle joint: Jiexi, Qiuxu, Kunlun.

捻挫傷

【弁症】

　局部がだるくて腫れ、疼痛し、或は少し赤く腫れ、運動が制限され、ひどくなると、転回できなくなる。

【治療】

処方：阿是穴。

症状による配穴：

　　頸項：天柱、後谿。

　　肩関節：肩井、肩髃。

　　肘関節：曲池、合谷。

　　腕関節：陽池、外関。

　　股関節：環跳、陽陵泉。

　　膝関節：犢鼻、内庭。

　　踝関節：解谿、丘墟、崑崙。

脏　躁

【辨证】

有各种神志异常见症，如无故悲伤，喜怒无常，多疑，善惊，心悸，烦躁，嗜眠不安等；或有突发胸闷，呃逆，暴瘖，抽搐等症。脉弦细。严重的可昏厥，僵仆。

【治疗】

处方：神门、三阴交。

随证配穴：胸闷：内关、膻中。

　　　　　呃逆：天突。

　　　　　暴瘖：廉泉、通里。

　　　　　抽搐：合谷、太冲。

　　　　　昏厥，僵仆：人中、涌泉。

Hysteria

【Differentiation】

Various psychotic symptoms such as melancholy without any assignable reason, paraphronia, suspiciousness, paraphobia, palpitation, irritability, somnolence, etc. There may be sudden onset of suffocating sensation, hiccup, aphonia and convulsion. The pulse is wiry and thready. In severe cases, there may be loss of consciousness and syncope.

【Treatment】

Prescription: Shenmen, Sanyinjiao.
Points according to different symptoms and signs:
Suffocating sensation: Neiguan, Shanzhong.
Hiccup: Tiantu.
Aphonia: Lianquan, Tongli.
Convulsion: Hegu, Taichong.
Loss of consciousness and syncope: Renzhong, Yongquan.

臟躁

【弁症】

いろいろな神志異常が見られ、例えば、理由もなしに悲しくなり、気うつりやすく、疑い深い。驚かされやすく、心悸、煩躁、嗜眠、不安などが見られる。或は急に胸が苦しくなり、しゃっくりしたり、急に聲が出なくなったり、痙攣などの症状が現

われる。脈は弦細である。甚しくなると，昏迷，僵撲（突然昏倒）する。

【治療】

処方：神門、三陰交。
症状による配穴：
　胸悶：内関、膻中。
　吃逆：天突。
　暴瘖：廉泉、通里。
　痙攣：合谷、太衝。
　昏迷、僵撲：人中、湧泉。

崩　　漏

【辨证】

经血忽然大下不止，称为血崩；持续不断称为漏下。两者常相互转变。一般症状有头目眩晕，精神疲倦，腰酸，四肢无力等。

血热：经色鲜红，有秽气，多兼烦躁，脉数，苔黄。
气虚：经色暗淡，少腹冷，多兼畏寒，面唇淡白，脉沉迟。

【治疗】

处方：关元、隐白。
随证配穴：血热：太冲。
　　　　　气虚：百会。

Uterine Hemorrhage

【Differentiation】

Uterine hemorrhage may be of abrupt onset, profuse or lingering and scanty, the two conditions possibly occur alternately. Other symptoms are dizziness, fatigue, low back pain and general weakness.

Heat in the blood: The blood is bright red with foul odour. Irritability, rapid pulse and yellow coated tongue are the common symptoms.

Deficiency of qi: The blood is pinkish and dull, there is cold sensation in the lower abdomen, usually with chilliness, pallor of the face and lips, deep slow pulse.

【Treatment】

Prescription: Guanyuan, Yinbai.
Points for different types:
Heat in the blood: Taichong.
Deficiency of qi: Baihui.

崩　　漏

【弁症】

突然に経血を大量排出して止まらないものを血崩と称し、たえずに流れ続くものを漏下と称する。両者は常に転化する。普通の症状は、眩暈、倦怠感、腰がだるく、四肢無力などである。

血熱：血の色が真赤で、いやなにおいがある。多くは煩躁を伴い、脈は数で、舌苔は黄色である。

気虚：血の色が暗くてうすく、下腹部が冷える。多くは寒がり、顔と唇の色が淡い。脈は沈遅である。

【治療】

処方：関元、隠白。

症状による配穴：

血熱：太衝。

気虚：百会。

痛　　经

【辨证】

实证：多在经前即开始少腹疼痛，痛的部位多固定不移，痛势剧烈，拒按，甚则牵引腰腿作痛，经来后痛渐减，经行不畅，色黑紫挟有瘀块，脉弦。

虚证：多在行经末期或经后少腹痛，痛势绵绵不休，得温暖与手按则缓，经色淡而少。甚者见形寒怕冷，心悸，头晕等症。

【治疗】

处方：

实证：中极、血海、合谷、三阴交。

虚证：关元、脾俞、肾俞、足三里、三阴交。

Dysmenorrhea

【Differentiation】

Shi type: Premenstrual cramping pain fixed in the lower abdomen and aggravated when pressed. This radiates to the lower back and thighs, gradually diminished after onset of menstruation; menstrual flow dark purple in colour with clots and with drainage difficulty; pulse wiry.

Xu type: Lower abdominal pain at late stage of menstruation or post-menstruation, mild but persistent pain responding to warmth and pressure, menstrual flow scanty and pink in colour. In severe cases, there may be chilliness, palpitation and dizziness. Pulse thready and forceless.

【Treatment】

Prescription:
Shi type: Zhongji, Xuehai, Hegu, Sanyinjiao.
Xu type: Guanyuan, Pishu, Shenshu, Zusanli, Sanyinjiao.

生理痛

【弁症】

実症：月経が来る前から下腹部が痛み始まり、痛みが激しく一定の所に固定し、押えることを拒む。甚しくなると腰や足まで痛くなる。月経が来てから痛みが次第に軽減する。月経の

量が少なく、色は黑紫で、瘀血の塊りを帯ぶ。脈は弦である。

虚症：多くは月経の後期あるいは月経後に下腹部が痛みが始まり、痛みは綿綿と続き、温めたり、手で押えたりしたら痛みがよくなる。血の色が淡く、量も少ない。ひどい場合には、寒がり、心悸、眩暈などが現われる。

【治療】

処方：

実症：中極、血海、合谷、三陰交。
虚症：関元、脾俞、腎俞、足三里、三陰交。

闭　　经

【辨证】

血滞：月经忽然停止，少腹胀痛，拒按，或有瘀块，脉沉弦。

血枯：经期后延，经量逐渐减少以至闭止，多有面色萎黄，皮肤干燥，精神不振，食少，便溏，苔白，脉无力。

【治疗】

处方：

血滞：中极、血海、三阴交、行间、合谷。
血枯：关元、肝俞、脾俞、肾俞、足三里、三阴交。

Amenorrhea

【Differentiation】

Blood stasis: Sudden onset, distention and pain in

the lower abdomen aggravated by pressure. There may be a mass on palpation. Deep wiry pulse.

Blood exhaustion: Delayed menstruation gradually decreasing in amount to amenorrhea, usually accompanied by sallow complexion, dry skin, listlessness, anorexia, loose stools, white coated tongue and forceless pulse.

【Treatment】

Prescription:
Blood stasis type: Zhongji, Xuehai, Sanyinjiao, Xingjian, Hegu.
Blood exhaustion type: Guanyuan, Ganshu, Pishu, Shenshu, Zusanli, Sanyinjiao.

月経閉止

【弁症】

血滞：急に月経閉止し、下腹部が膨満して痛む。押さえられるのを拒み、あるいは血に塊りがあり、脈は沈弦である。

血枯：月経の周期が後延し、量も少しずつ減り、ついに停止する。顔色は黄色になり、皮膚が乾燥し、精神的に倦怠する。食欲不振、大便が流動状軟便を排出する。舌苔は白く、脈は無力である。

【治療】

処方：
血滞：中極、血海、三陰交、行間、合谷。
血枯：関元、肝兪、脾兪、腎兪、足三里、三陰交。

带　下

【辨证】

带下有白带，黄带之分。因气虚夹湿的，其色白而稀薄或淡黄，有腥臊气，称为白带；因湿热下注的，其色多淡红或深黄，腥臭难闻，称为黄带。常有腰酸，头晕，肢体倦怠等症。

【治疗】

处方：带脉、气海、三阴交。
随证配穴：白带：肾俞、关元、足三里。
　　　　　黄带：中极、阴陵泉、行间。

Leukorrhea

【Differentiation】

Leukorrhea may be differentiated as white or yellow discharge.

White discharge is due to insufficiency of qi and presence of damp. It is thin, whitish or yellowish, with odour.

Yellow discharge is due to downward infusion of damp-heat. It is pink or deep yellow with fetid odour.

Both conditions may be accompanied by low back pain, dizziness and lassitude.

【Treatment】

Prescription: Daimai, Qihai, Sanyinjiao.
Points for different symptoms:
White discharge: Shenshu, Guanyuan, Zusanli.
Yellow discharge: Zhongji, Yinlingquan, Xingjian.

帯　下

【弁症】

　帯下には白帯と黄帯との区別がある。気虚の上に湿邪をはさむ場合は、その色が白くて薄いか淡黄色で生臭い。これを白帯という。湿熱下注の場合は色が淡紅色あるいは濃黄色で、いやな生臭いにおいがあり、これを黄帯という。腰がだるく、眩暈、倦怠無力などの症状を伴う。

【治療】

　処方：帯脈、気海、三陰交。
　症状による配穴：
　　白帯：腎兪、関元、足三里。
　　黄帯：中極、陰陵泉、行間。

妊娠悪阻

【辨証】

　怀孕月余之后，即开始有恶心呕吐，或食入即吐，甚至见到饮食或嗅到气味即引起呕吐，兼见心胸烦满，头晕，目眩，四肢倦怠等症。

【治疗】

处方：足三里、内关、上脘。

Morning Sickness

【Differentiation】

Nausea and vomiting occur after about one month of pregnancy. Vomiting may take place right after food intake or at the sight or smell of food. The accompanying symptoms are fullness in chest, dizziness, blurring of vision and lassitude.

【Treatment】

Prescription: Zusanli, Neiguan Shangwan.

妊娠悪阻

【弁症】

妊娠して一個月余りから、噁心、嘔吐が始まり、或は食べ次第に吐き出し、甚しくなると、飲食物を見るだけて、または嗅ぐだけて嘔吐する。心胸煩満、眩暈、四肢無力などの症状を兼ねて見る。

【治療】

処方：足三里、内関、上脘。

胎位不正

【辨证】

胎位不正是指妊娠30周后，胎儿在子宫体内的位置不正，常见于经产妇或腹壁松弛的孕妇。产妇本身多无自觉症状。产科检查后明确诊断如臀位、横位等。

【治疗】

处方：至阴。

方法：操作时须解松腰带，坐在靠背椅上或仰卧床上，以艾条灸两侧至阴穴15～20分钟，每天1～2次，至胎位转正为止。据报道成功率达80%。对骨盆狭窄，子宫畸形引起者，应作其他处理。

Abnormal Position of Fetus

【Differentiation】

This means the fetus is in an abnormal position in the uterus after thirty weeks of pregnancy. It is often seen in multipara or pregnant women who have laxity of the abdominal wall. The pregnant woman herself has no subjective symptoms and precise diagnosis is confirmed by the breech position or transverse position on obstetric examination.

【Treatment】

Prescription: Zhiyin.

Method: The patient sits on a chair or lies down on her back on the bed. The belt should be loosen during manipulation. Moxa sticks are used for Zhiyin points on both sides and for 15〜20 minutes. This is done once or twice a day until the position of the fetus is normal. It is reported that the rate of success has reached 80%. We should use other procedure when this problem is due to a narrow pelvis or abnormality of the uterus.

胎位不正

【弁症】

胎位不正とは、妊娠30週間後、胎児の子宮内の位置が正常でないことを指す。経産婦あるいは腹壁のゆるんでいる妊婦に多く見られる。妊婦は、自覚症状がないことが多く、産婦人科の診察によって、正確に診断されるものである。例えば、殿位、横位など。

【治療】

処方：至陰。

方法：操作する時は、まず患者のバンドをゆるめ、背のある椅子に坐らせるか床の上に仰臥させ、艾条で両側の至陰穴を15〜20分間灸する。1日に1〜2回で、胎児の位置が正常になるまで続ける。報告によると、その成功率は80%に達する。骨盤狭窄と子宮の奇形により起されたものは、ほかの措置を考えなければならない。

乳 汁 少

【辨证】

产后乳汁分泌不足，甚至点滴不下，或哺乳期中日见减少。如兼见心悸，神疲，乳汁清稀，属虚证。如兼见胸闷食少，乳汁不行，胁痛等，属实证。

【治疗】

处方：乳根、膻中、少泽。
随证配穴：虚证：脾俞、足三里。
　　　　　实证：内关、期门。

Lactation Insufficiency

【Differentiation】

Scanty or absence of milk secretion after childbirth, or continuous decrease in quantity during lactation. In the xu type, the accompanying symptoms are palpitation, lassitude and thin milk. In the shi type, there appear fullness in chest, anorexia, retention of milk and hypochondriac pain.

【Treatment】

Prescription: Rugen, Shanzhong, Shaoze.
Secondary points:
Xu type: Pishu, Zusanli.
Shi type: Neiguan, Qimen.

乳汁分泌不足

【弁症】

　分娩した後、乳汁の分泌が不足し、甚しい時は、一滴も分泌しない。あるいは哺乳期において、乳汁の分泌が日ましに減少する。心悸、倦怠感があり、乳汁が稀薄であれば、虚症に属し、胸部苦悶感、食欲不振、乳汁が流れ出ず、側胸部疼痛などがあれば、実症に属する。

【治療】

　処方：乳根、膻中、少沢。
　症状による配穴：
　　　虚症：脾俞、足三里。
　　　実症：内関、期門。

小儿惊风

【辨证】

　急惊风：高热昏厥，两目上视，口噤不开，痰涎壅盛，手足抽搐，角弓反张，面现青紫色，脉弦数。
　慢惊风：形体消瘦，面色㿠白，神疲，昏睡露睛，时而抽搐，四肢清冷，大便溏薄或完谷不化，小便清长，脉沉弱无力。

【治疗】

　处方：十宣、印堂、人中、曲池、太冲。

随证配穴：昏厥不醒：劳宫、涌泉。
抽搐不止：行间、阳陵泉、昆仑、后溪。
发热不退：大椎、合谷。

Infantile Convulsion

【Differentiation】

Acute convulsion: High fever, coma, upward staring eyes, clenched jaws, rattles, tetanic contraction, opisthotonos, cyanosis, rapid and wiry pulse.

Chronic convulsion: Emaciation, pallor, lassitude, lethargy with half-closed eyes, intermittent convulsion, cold extremities, loose stools with undigested food, profuse clear urine, deep feeble pulse.

【Treatment】

Prescription: Shixuan, Yintang, Renzhong, Quchi, Taichong.

Secondary points for different symptoms and signs: Coma: Laogong, Yongquan.

Protracted convulsion: Xingjian, Yanglingquan, Kunlun, Houxi.

Continuous high fever: Dazhui, Hegu.

小児驚風

【弁証】

急驚風：高熱、昏迷、両眼が上視し、歯をかたく閉じ、痰と涎沫の分泌が盛んで、手足が攣急し、後弓反張、顔はチアノ

ーゼを現わす。脈は弦数である。

慢驚風：体形が瘦せ、顔色は蒼白く、倦怠感があり、目を閉じないで昏睡し、たまたま攣急して、四肢が冷え、大便は流動状軟便あるいは未消化物を排泄し、小便は清らかで長い。脈は沈弱無力である。

【治療】

処方：十宣、印堂、人中、曲池、太衝。

症状による配穴：

目がさめないで昏迷するものは：勞宮、湧泉。

攣急が引続いておこる場合は：行間、陽陵泉、崑崙、後谿。

熱が下がらない場合は：大椎、合谷。

小 儿 腹 泻

【辨证】

腹胀肠鸣，时时作痛，痛则欲泻，泻后痛缓；1日可泻几次或十几次，泻物酸腐臭秽，或有乳谷不化，频作嗳气，不思食，舌苔腻，脉沉而少力。

【治疗】

处方：中脘、天枢、上巨虚、四缝。

随证配穴：外感寒邪加合谷。

Infantile Diarrhea

【Dfferentiation】

Abdominal distension, borborygmus, intermittent abdominal pain relieved after diarrhea which may occur from several to more than ten times a day with strong fetid odour and at times producing stools mixed with milk curd, frequent belching, anorexia. Tongue is sticky coated, pulse deep and forceless.

【Treatment】

Prescription: Zhongwan, Tianshu, Shangjuxu, Sifeng.
Secondary points:
Exogenous cold: Hegu.

小児下痢

【弁症】

腹部膨満、腸鳴、たまたま腹痛し、痛み次第に排便したく、排出すると痛みが緩解する。1日数回乃至十数回も排便し、排泄物は酸敗して臭く、あるいは乳汁未消化便、時時噯気、食欲不振。舌苔は膩で、脈は沈かつ無力である。

【治療】

処方：中脘、天枢、上巨虚、四縫。
症状による配穴：
　　寒邪に侵された場合：合谷を加える。

耳鸣耳聋

【辨证】

实证：耳鸣是鸣声不止，按之不减。耳聋系骤然致聋。多兼有头胀重，鼻塞，口苦，胁痛，苔腻，脉滑数。

虚证：耳鸣时作时止，过劳加剧，按之鸣声稍减。耳聋是渐次增重。多兼头昏眼花，腰脊酸痛，神倦，脉细。

【治疗】

处方：翳风、耳门、听会、中渚、听宫。
随证配穴：实证：行间、足临泣、外关。
　　　　　虚证：肾俞、太溪、三阴交。

Deafness and Tinnitus

【Differentiation】

Shi type:
Tinnitus: Continuous ringing of the ear unrelieved by pressure.
Deafness: Sudden deafness.
The accompanying symptoms and signs are distension and heavy sensation of the head, nasal obstruction, bitter taste in mouth, hypochondriac pain, sticky coated tongue and rolling rapid pulse.

Xu type:
Tinnitus: Intermittent ringing of the ear which becomes aggravated after stress and strain and is some-

what alleviated by pressure.

Deafness: Gradually intensified deafness.

The accompanying symptoms and signs are dizziness, blurring of vision, low back pain, lassitude and thready pulse.

【Treatment】

Prescription: Yifeng, Ermen, Tinghui, Zhongzhu, Tinggong.

Secondary points:
Shi type: Xingjian, Foot-Linqi, Waiguan.
Xu type: Sheshu, Taixi, Sanyinjiao.

耳鳴、難聴

【弁症】

実症:耳鳴は、耳の中でたえまなく鳴きこえがし、耳を押えても軽減しない。難聴は発病が突然である（暴聾）。多くは、頭が重く、鼻がつまり、口が苦く、側胸痛などが見られ、舌苔は膩で、脈は滑数である。

虚症:耳鳴がしたり、絶えたりし、疲労した時など特にひどくなり、押えると鳴きこえがやや軽減する。難聴では、発病が比較的緩慢なものである。多くは、めまい、頭昏、腰がだるくて痛み、倦怠感があり、脈は細である。

【治療】

処方:翳風、耳門、聴会、中渚、聴宮。
症状による配穴:
　　実症:行間、足臨泣、外関。

虚症：肾俞、太豁、三阴交。

目赤肿痛

【辨证】

目赤肿痛，灼热怕光，流泪眵多，兼有头痛，发热，脉浮数者为风热；兼有口苦，烦热，大便秘结，脉弦者，为肝胆火旺。

【治疗】

处方：合谷、睛明、风池、太阳、行间。
随证配穴：肝胆火旺加太冲、光明。

Congestion, Swelling and Pain of the Eye

【Differentiation】

Congestion, swelling, pain and burning sensation of the eye, photophobia, lacrimation and sticky discharge.

Invasion of exogenous wind-heat: Headache, fever, superficial rapid pulse.

Upward disturbance of fire of liver and gall bladder: Bitter taste in mouth, irritability with feverish sensation, constipation, wiry pulse.

【Treatment】

Prescription: Hegu, Jingming, Fengchi, Taiyang, Xingjian.

Secondary points:

Upward disturbance of fire of liver and gall bladder: Taichong, Guangming.

目赤腫痛

【弁症】

　目が赤く腫れて痛み、灼熱感があって、羞明し、流涙と分泌物が増加する。頭痛、発熱などを伴う、脈が浮数であるものは風熱であり、口が苦く、煩熱があって、大便秘結、脈が弦であるものは肝胆火旺（肝胆の火が激しい）である。

【治療】

　処方：合谷、睛明、風池、太陽、行間。
　症状による配穴：
　　　肝胆火旺のものには：太衝、光明を加える。

齿 痛

【辨证】

　风热：牙龈肿痛，口渴喜冷饮，大便秘结，舌质红苔黄，脉数。
　肾虚：绵绵作痛，牙齿浮动，时痛时止，舌质红，脉细数。

【治疗】

　处方：颊车、下关。
　随证配穴：风热：合谷、内庭、风池。
　　　　　　肾虚：太溪。

Toothache

【Differentiation】

Wind-heat: Gingival swelling and pain, thirst and preference for cold beverages, constipation, red tongue with yellow coating, rapid pulse.

Xu of kidney: Intermittent dull pain, loose teeth, red tongue, thready rapid pulse.

【Treatment】

Prescription: Jiache, Xiaguan.
Points according to symptoms:
Wind-heat: Hegu, Neiting, Fengchi.
Xu of kidney: Taixi.

歯痛

【弁症】

風熱：歯齦腫痛、口渇があり、つめたいものを飲みたい。大便は秘結し、舌質が赤く、舌苔は黄色、脈は数である。

腎虚：綿綿と痛みが続き、歯が浮き、痛みが出たり消えたり、舌質が赤く、脈は細数てある。

【治療】

処方：頬車、下関。
症状による配穴：
　　風熱：合谷、内庭、風池。
　　腎虚：太谿。

咽喉肿痛

【辨证】

实证：起病急骤，恶寒发热，头痛，咽喉肿痛，口渴，便秘，舌红，苔薄黄，脉浮数。

虚证：起病缓慢，无热或低热，咽喉时痛时止，咽干，入夜较重，手足心热，舌红无苔，脉细数。

【治疗】

处方：实证：少商、合谷、内庭、天容。
　　　虚证：太溪、列缺、鱼际、照海。

Sore Throat

【Differentiation】

Shi type: Abrupt onset with a chill, fever and headache, congested and sore throat, thirst, constipation, red tongue with thin yellow coating, superficial rapid pulse.

Xu type: Gradual onset without fever or with low fever, intermittent sore throat, dryness of the throat which usually becomes aggravated by night, feverish sensation in palms and soles, uncoated red tongue, thready rapid pulse.

【Treatment】

Prescription:
Shi type: Shaoshang, Hegu, Neiting, Tianrong,

Xu type: Taixi, Lieque, Yuji, Zhaohai.

咽喉腫痛

【弁症】

実症：発病が突然で、悪寒発熱、頭痛、咽喉腫痛、口渇、便秘などがあり、舌質が赤く、舌苔は薄く黄色、脈は浮数である。

虚症：発病が緩慢で、平熱もしくは微熱。咽喉の痛みがあったりなくなったり、舌質が赤く、舌苔がなく、脈は細数である。

【治療】

処方：実症：少商、合谷、内庭、天容。
　　　虚症：太谿、列缺、魚際、照海。

鼻衄

【辨证】

肺胃热盛：伴有发热，咳嗽，口渴，便秘,脉浮数等。
阴虚火旺：伴有颧红，口干，手脚心热，甚或午后潮热，脉细数等。

【治疗】

处方：合谷、上星。
随证配穴：肺热：少商。
　　　　　胃热：内庭。
　　　　　阴虚火旺：太溪。

Epistaxis

【Differentiation】

Excess of heat in lung and stomach: Epistaxis is accompanied by fever, cough, thirst, constipation and superficial rapid pulse.

Hyperactivity of fire due to insufficiency of yin: Epistaxis is accompanied by malar flush, dryness of mouth and feverish sensation in palms and soles. In severe cases there may be afternoon fever and thready rapid pulse.

【Treatment】

Prescription: Hegu, Shangxing.
Secondary points:
Heat of the lung: Shaoshang.
Heat of the stomach: Neiting.
Hyperactivity of fire due to insufficiency of yin: Taixi.

鼻　血

【弁症】

　肺胃熱盛：発熱、咳嗽、口渇、便秘などを伴う。脈は浮数である。
　陰虚火旺：顔がほてり、口乾、手掌と足底に熱感があり、甚しくなると、午後には潮熱があり、脈は細数である。

【治療】

処方：合谷、上星。
症状による配穴：
　　肺熱：少商。
　　胃熱：内庭。
　　陰虚火旺：太谿。

风　疹

【辨证】

风疹发作迅速。瘙痒异常，皮肤出现大小不一疹块，或兼有腹痛，大便秘结，脉多浮数。急性者消退亦快，慢性者常见反复发作。

【治疗】

处方：血海、三阴交、曲池、合谷。
随证配穴：腹痛加足三里。

【参考】

本病相当于荨麻疹。

Urticaria

【Differentiation】

Abrupt onset with itching wheals of various size. There may be accompanying abdominal pain, constipation and superficial rapid pulse. Acute conditions subside quickly, while recurrences are frequent when the disease is chronic.

【Treatment】

Prescription: Xuehai, Sanyinjiao, Quchi, Hegu.
Secondary points:
Abdominal pain: Zusanli.

風　疹

【弁症】

風疹は急に発作する。非常に掻痒感があり、皮膚にさまざまな大きさの丘疹が現われ、或は腹痛、便秘を兼ね、脈は多く浮数である。急性発作の者は丘疹の消失も速く、慢性の者は、常に繰返して発作する。

【治療】

処方：血海、三陰交、曲池、合谷。
症状による配穴：
　　腹痛には：足三里を加える。

【参考】

本症は蕁麻疹にあたる。

缠腰火丹

【辨证】

发生于腰际侧肋之间，有小水疱如联珠状，簇聚成行，灼痛

异常，皮肤红热。

【治疗】

处方：曲池、血海、委中、夹脊穴（可在发病部位沿肋骨水平取夹脊穴。）

【参考】

相当现代医学带状疱疹。

Herpes Zoster

【Differentiation】

Herpes zoster occurs mainly in the lumbar and hypochondriac regions, with small vesicles like beads forming a girdle. Severe burning pain and redness and hotness of the skin mark the disease.

【Treatment】

Prescription: Quchi, Xuehai, Weizhong. Huatuo Jiaji points (corresponding to the site of lesion is also advisable).

纆腰火丹

【弁症】

腰肋間に発生し、小さい水疱が出て、累累と数珠のように束帯状にならぶ。非常に灼痛し、皮膚が赤くて熱い。

【治療】

处方：曲池、血海、委中。

夾脊穴（発病部位で肋骨に沿って水平する夾脊穴を刺してよい）。

【参考】

現代医学の帯状疱疹にあたる。

疔　　疮

【辨证】

疔疮有发于头面的，也有生于手足的。初起状如米粒，形小根硬，或痛或麻，或起水疱、脓疱，黄紫不一，坚着如钉，多有恶寒发热。

【治疗】

处方：灵台、身柱、合谷、委中。

【参考】

本病亦可采用挑治，即寻找背部脊柱两旁有丘疹样突起处，用粗针挑治，每日1次。

Furuncle

【Differentiation】

Furuncle may occur on the head, face or extremities. It first appears like a grain of millet, with a hard base. Pain or a tingling sensation may be present. A blister or pustula yellowish or purplish in colour and hard as a nail is formed, usually accompanied by chills and fever.

【Treatment】

Prescription: Lingtai, Shenzhu, Hegu, Weizhong.

【Remark】

Pricking and tilting with the thick needle may be used to treat this disease. That is, to find the small papules which may appear alongside the thoracic vertebrae. Treatment may be given once a day.

疔瘡

【弁症】

疔瘡は、顔面に発生するものもあれば、四肢に発生するものもある。発症の初期は、皮膚に米粒のような小さくて硬いものができ、痛みまたはしびれ、あるいは水疱、膿疱ができ、黄色または紫色で、釘のようにかたくつけ、多くは悪寒発熱がある。

【治療】

処方：霊台、身柱、合谷、委中。

【参考】

三稜針でつきやぶって治療する。脊柱の両側にできる小さい丘疹を毎日1回つきやぶっても、疔瘡に一定の治効がある。

气　　瘿

【辨证】

颈部肿大，有的兼有胸膈气闷，心悸气促，眼球突出，暴躁善怒，脉象弦滑等。

【治疗】

处方：天突、翳风、合谷、丰隆。
随证配穴：肝郁气滞：膻中、太冲。
　　　　　眼球突出：风池、睛明、太阳。
　　　　　　　　　可在颈部肿大处取穴。

【参考】

相当现代医学甲状腺机能亢进、甲状腺肿等。

Goiter

【Differentiation】

Swelling of the neck, which may be accompanied by stuffiness in the chest, palpitation, shortness of breath, exophthalmos and irascibility. Pulse is wiry and rolling.

【Treatment】

Prescription: Tiantu, Yifeng, Hegu, Fenglong.
Secondary points:
Depression of qi of Liver: Shanzhong, Taichong.
Exophthalmos: Fengchi, Jingming, Taiyang. Points

may be selected in the area of swelling of the neck.

【Remark】

Goiter as described in this section corresponds to hyperthyroidism and goiter of modern medicine.

気　瘿

【弁症】

頸部が腫大し、ある場合には胸が重苦しく、心悸亢進、呼吸がせわしくなる。眼球突出、怒りっぽくなるなどの症がある。脈は弦滑である。

【治療】

処方：天突、翳風、合谷、豊隆。

症状による配穴：

　　　肝気うっ結の場合：膻中、太衝。

　　　眼球突出の場合：風池、晴明、太陽。頸部の腫大したところに穴を取ってもよい。

【参考】

本症は現代医学の単純性甲状腺腫、バセドー氏病にあたる。

消 渴

【辨证】

上消：口渴多饮或虚痨咳嗽，皮肤干燥或疮疡。
中消：消谷善饥，或有自汗，气短，面白，肢冷等。
下消：小便频数，尿量增多，腰部疼痛等。

【治疗】

处方：上消：鱼际、复溜。
　　　中消：中脘、足三里、照海。
　　　下消：关元、带脉、三阴交。
　　　热盛脉大：曲池、支沟、阳陵泉、足三里。

【参考】

相当现代医学糖尿病、尿崩症等。

Emaciation-Thirst Diseases

【Differentiation】

Shangxiao (The upper emaciation): Polydipsia or cough due to asthenia of viscera, dry skin or pyogenic infection and ulcerous disease of the skin.

Zhongxiao (The middle emaciation): Polyorexia or spontaneous perspiration, shortness of breath, pallor and cold extremities.

Xiaxiao (The lower emaciation): Frequency of micturition, polyuria, low back pain.

【Treatment】

Prescription:

Shangxiao(The upper emaciation): Yuji, Fuliu.

Zhongxiao (The middle emaciation): Zhongwan, Zusanli, Zhaohai.

Xiaxiao(The lower emaciation): Guanyuan, Daimai, Sanyinjiao.

Excessive heat and a forceful pulse: Quchi, Zhigou, Yanglingquan, Zusanli.

【Remark】

This is equivalent to diabetes mellitus, and diabetes insipidus of advanced medicine.

消　　渇

【弁症】

上消：口が渇き水物を多くとる。咳、皮膚乾燥あるいは腫瘍または潰瘍を発する。

中消：多く食べても空腹感を覚え、かえって体が痩せ衰え、汗が知らぬ間に外に流出する。気短、顔色が白く、四肢が冷えるなどの症がある。

下消：小便頻数、尿の量も多い。腰部疼痛などの症がある。

【治療】

処方：上消：魚際、復溜。

中消：中脘、足三里、照海。
下消：関元、帯脈、三陰交。
熱盛脈大：曲池，支溝，陽陵泉，足三里。

【参考】

現代医学の糖尿病、尿崩症などにあたる。

【附】典型病例介绍
【Appendix】 Examples of Typical Cases
【附】症例解説

例1：针刺3次，完全控制持续不止的呃逆。

纪××，男，62岁，住院号181721。

主诉：持续不止呃逆半天。

现病史：患者因患"急性心肌梗塞"在内科住院。半天前突发呃逆，持续不止，而请针灸科会诊。

查体：表情苦闷，呃逆持续不止，呃声较大，舌胖且有齿痕，苔白，脉沉弦。

诊断：呃逆。

治疗经过：取内关、足三里、天突、中脘，针后即好转，继续巩固治疗3次，呃逆得以完全控制。

Example 1: A case of continuous hiccup completely controled by three acupuncture treatments.

Ji ××, Male, Age 62, Case No 181721.

Chief Complaint: Continuous hiccup for a half day.

History of Illness: The patient was admitted to the internal medicine department with "acute myocardial infarction". The onset of hiccup occurred suddenly and continuously for a half day. The department of acupuncture and moxibustion was consulted.

Physical Examination: The patient was despondent and depressed with continuous and load hiccup. The tongue was swollen with teeth-marks on its edges, and was white coated. The pulse was deep and wiry.

Diagnosis: Hiccup.

Treatment: Selected points are Neiguan, Zusanli, Tiantu, Zhongwan, etc. The conditions became better as soon as acupuncture had been given. Repetition of treatment three times completely controled the hiccup.

例1：3回の針療法で，持続して止まらないしゃっくりを完全におさえる。

紀××、男、62才、住院番號181721。

主訴：半日間しゃっくりが持続して止まらない。

現病歷：患者は、急性心筋梗塞症で内科に住院しているもので、半日前から突然しゃっくりが始まり、持続して止まらないため、針灸科の診察を求めた。

檢査：表情が苦んで、しゃっくりが持続して止まらない、音も比較的大きい。舌が肥大し、かつ歯痕があり、舌苔は白く、脈は沈弦であった。

診斷：吃逆（しゃっくり）。

治療経過：内関、足三里、天突、中脘などの穴を取り、針を刺した後すぐ好転した。その後、続いて3回治療して、しゃっくりが完全にとまった。

例2：治疗4次，持续2个月的三叉神经痛痊愈。

宋××，女，52岁。

主诉：右面部剧烈灼痛已2个月。

现病史：2个月前生气后，诱发右侧面部剧烈灼痛，呈阵发性，1次约1小时，严重时1日发作4～5次。经神经科诊为"三叉神经痛"。曾服用中、西药均未控制，1982年2月8日来门诊求治。

诊断：右三叉神经痛（Ⅰ、Ⅱ、Ⅲ支）。

治疗经过：取右侧太阳、下关、颊车，用0.85%盐水2～4ml行穴位注射，痛即好转。治疗4次，完全治愈。

Example2: Continually persisted trigeminal neuralgia for two months cured by four acupuncture treatments.

Song ××, Female, Age 52.

Chief Complaint: Badly burning pain on the right face for two months.

History of Illness: Badly burning pain on the right face apparently induced after anger two months previously, the attack continued for about an hour and may occur 4～5 times a day when the condition became severe. "Trigeminal neuralgia" was diagnosed by the neurologist. The patient had used traditional Chinese medicine and western medicine, but the condition was not controlled. The patient came to the out-patient department for treatment on February 8, 1982.

Diagnosis: Right trigeminal neuralgia (Ⅰ.Ⅱ.Ⅲ.branches).

Treatment: Selected points of Taiyang, Xiaguan, Jiache on the right side. On injecting into these points with 0.85% saline, the pain became less. The patient was completely cured after four treatments.

例2　4回の治療で、2个月もつらなった三叉神経痛が治癒。

宋××、女、52才。

主訴：2个月前から右側顔面が激しく灼痛。

現病歴：2个月前に腹をたてた時、右側顔面部の激しい灼痛を誘発。発作性で、毎回約1時間。甚しい時は、1日に4～5回発作する。神経科で「三叉神経痛」と診断されたが、漢方薬と西洋薬を服用しても改善がみられないので、1982年2月8日に外来で、針灸治療を求めた。

診断：右三叉神経痛（Ⅰ、Ⅱ、Ⅲ枝）。

治療経過：右側の太陽、下関、頬車などの穴を取り、0.85％のNaClを2～4ml穴位に注射して、痛みがすぐ改善され、4回の治療で、完全に治癒した。

例3：术后排尿困难，针治2次，效果显著。

刘××，女，49岁，住院号109448。

主诉：手术后排尿困难已4天。

现病史：4天前，病人因"胆结石"行外科手术，术后即出现排尿困难，已行留置导尿术4天。

治疗经过：取中极、横骨、三阴交，针刺后即能主动排出少量尿液。次日复取次髎、肾俞、秩边、长强等穴，针刺后即能拔出导管，自主排尿。

Example 3: Dysuria postoperatively. After two acupuncture treatments, the improvement was marked.

Liu××, Female, Age 49, Case No 109448.

Chief Complaint: Four days of difficulty in passing water following an operation.

History of Illness: The patient had been operated for gallstone four days previously, and dysuria occurred just after the operation. Catheterization had been carried out for four days.

Treatment: Zhongji, Henggu, Sanyinjiao were taken. A small urinary output could be produced after acupuncture. Ciliao, Shenshu, Zhibian, Changqiang, etc. were also taken the next day. The catheter was withdrawn after acupuncture and voluntary urination was established.

例3：術後排尿困難、針治療2回で、顕著な効果を収めた。

劉××、女、49才、住院番号109448。

主訴：手術後排尿困難となり、4日目である。

現病歴：4日前、患者は、胆石症のため外科手術を受けた。術後排尿困難となり、留置カテーテルをして、4日目である。

治療経過：中極、横骨、三陰交などの穴を取り、針刺した後少量の尿液を自主排出した。翌日は、次髎、腎俞、秩辺、長強などの穴を取り、針刺した後、カテーテルを取り出し、自主排尿することができた。

例4：针刺治疗1个月，使膀胱造瘘8年的病人自主排尿。

崔××，男，26岁，住院号190968。

主诉：因尿潴留行膀胱造瘘已8年。

现病史：患者从6岁开始滴尿、遗尿，18岁时出现排尿困难，经北京

某医院诊断为"尿道内息肉阻塞性尿潴留"而行膀胱造瘘术，术后仍排尿困难，故来院要求针灸治疗。

查体：骶尾部有一小隐窝，骶神经4～5区感觉障碍。舌淡，苔白，尺脉弱。X光拍片显示骶一椎体有裂。

诊断：癃闭（先天性骶椎裂引起尿潴留）。

治疗经过：取秩边、会阴、中极、三阴交等穴，每日针刺1次，计30次，完全恢复自主排尿，并拔掉造瘘管。

1年后随访疗效巩固。

Example 4: A patient who had cystofistulation eight years earlier could urinate voluntaryly after one month of acupuncture treatment.

Cui×× , Male, Age 26, Case No 190968.

Chief Complaint: The patient had undergone cystofistulation eight years earlier because of retention of urine.

History of Illness: The patient had suffered from urine dribb-le and enuresis since he was six years old. At the age of eightfieen, he began to suffer from dysuria."Obstructive retention o urine because of polypus in urethra"was diagnosed by certain hospital in Beijing. The patient underwent cystofistulation but after the operation dysuria recurred. The patient then came to our hospital and accepted acupuncture treatment.

Physical Examination: There was a small crypt in the sacral caudal region and sensory disturbance in the regions corresponding to the nerves of the 4th and 5th sacral vertibrae. The Tongue was pale and white-coated. The pulse was weak, especially at the proximal part. An x-ray film showed sacral spina bifida.

Diagnosis: Retention of urine(due to congenital sacral spina bifida).

Treatment: Selected points of Zhibian, Huiyin, Zhongji, Sanyinjiao, etc. Acupuncture once a day. Voluntary urination regainef completely and the catheter was then taken out after a total do thirty acupuncture treatments.

When a follow-up was made after a year, the therapeutic response remained the same as on discharge.

例4： 針療法1个月で、膀胱瘻設置術8年の患者が自主排尿できた。

崔××、男、26才、住院番号190968.

主訴：尿閉で膀胱瘻設置術を受けて8年。

現病歴：患者は、6才から滴尿と遺尿を始め、18才に排尿困難が現われ、北京の病院で、尿路ポリープ閉塞性尿閉と診断され、膀胱瘻設置術を受けた。術後なお排尿困難が続き、針灸治療を求めに来た。

検査：尾骶部に小さい隠窩が一つあり、骶神経の4～5区に感覚障害を有す。舌がうすく、舌苔が白い。脈は尺脈が弱であった。レントゲンでは骶骨の第一椎体に裂痕があらわれていた。

診断：尿閉（先天性骶椎裂）。

治療経過：秩辺、会陰、中極、三陰交などの穴を取り、毎日1回針刺し、30回で自主排尿を完全に回復した。カテーテルを取り除いた。

1年後に訪問した時、治療効果は持続していた。

例5： 针刺治疗急性膀胱炎，疗效快而好。

王××，女，49岁，住院号171502。

主诉：尿频、尿急已2天。

现病史：病人体质素弱，2天前劳累后，出现尿频、尿急，并伴有下腹部坠胀感、腰痛、无发冷发热。因用西药过敏而要求中医治疗。

查体：膀胱区有压痛，舌淡红，苔白，脉弦。查尿常规：蛋白(++)、白细胞10～24/400x、红细胞10～30/400x。

诊断：淋证（急性膀胱炎）。

治疗经过：取中极、肾俞、三阴交、足三里等穴，每日1次，3次后症状消失，6次后尿常规检查恢复正常出院。

1年后随访疗效巩固。

Example 5: Acute cystitis was treated with acupuncture. The result was favourable and rapid.

Wang××, Female, Age 49, Case No 171502.

Chief Complaint: Frequency and urgency of micturition for two days.

History of Illness: Patient's general condition had been poor. Two days previously, frequency and urgency had occurred accompanied by a feeling of sinking in the lower part of the abdomen after over-fatigue. She suffered from lower back pain with no sensation of cold or heat there. The patient requested traditional Chinese medicine for treatment because she was allergic to western medicine.

Physical Examination : There was tenderness in the bladder area, a pink white-coated tongue, and wiry pulse. Standard laboratory urine examination showed: albumin (++), white blood cell counts 10~24/400x, red blood cell counts 10~30/400x.

Diagnosis: Stranguria(Acute cystitis).

Treatment: Selected points of Zhongji, Shenshu, Sanyinjiao, Zusanli, etc. once a day. The symptoms disappeared after three treatments. Examination of urine showed a return to normal after six acupuncture treatments. The patient was discharged from the hospital.

The steady result was found to have been maintained when a follow-up was made after a year.

例5：針で急性膀胱炎を治療するには、効果がはやく、たいへんよい方法である。

王××、女、49オ、住院番号171502。

主訴：尿意頻数、尿意切迫で2日。

現病歴：病人の体質が弱く、2日前過労した後、尿意頻数と尿意切迫の感じが現われ、下腹部の堕脹感を伴う、腰痛があり、発熱と悪寒はない。西洋薬にアナフィラキシーがあるので、漢方治療を求めた。

検査：膀胱区に圧痛がある。舌はうすあかく、舌苔は白く、脈は弦であった。尿検査では、蛋白(++)WBC 10~24/400x, RBC10~30/400x。

診断：淋症（急性膀胱炎）

治療経過：中極、腎俞、三陰交、足三里などの穴を取り、毎日1回刺し、3回後に症状がなくなり、6回後に尿検査の結果が全部正常に回復して退院した。

1年後に訪問した時、治療の効果がなお持続していた。

例6：针刺治疗坐骨神经痛，效果显著。
赵××，男，26岁。
主诉：右下肢剧烈疼痛已3天。
现病史：病人3天前遇凉后，右腿疼痛、不能持重，活动受限。经神经科诊断为"坐骨神经痛"。要求针灸治疗。
查体：Lasegue's氏征（+），苔白，脉弦。
诊断：痹证（坐骨神经痛）。
治疗经过：取环跳、阳陵泉、足三里、昆仑等穴（其中环跳穴，1次注入0.85%盐水20ml），治疗后，疼痛立止，并能站立行走。针治7次后痊愈。

Example 6: A favourable result was obtainned with acupuncture treatment for sciatica.
Zhao××, Male, Age 26.
Chief Complaint: Severe pain in the right leg for three days.
History of Illness: After the patient was exposed to cold weather three days previously, the right leg was painful and could not hold his weight. The leg action was limited. "Sciatic neuralgia" was diagnosed by the doctors in Neurology and Psychiatry Department. Acupuncture treatment was requested.
Physical Examination: Lasegue's syndrome(+), white-coated tongue, and wiry pulse.
Diagnosis: Bi syndrome (sciatic neuralgia).
Treatment: Selected points of Huantiao. Yanglingquan. Zusanli, Kunlun etc. 20ml of 0.85% saline was injected once into the Huantiao point. The pain stopped immediately after injection. The patient could stand and walk, and completely recovered after seven acupuncture treatments.

例6 針刺療法は、坐骨神経痛に効果顕著。
趙××、男、26才。
主訴：右下肢が激しく痛んで3日間。
現病歴：3日前に患者は冷えにあたり、右下肢に痛みを感じ、体重

をささえることができなくなり、歩行も制限され、神経科で「坐骨神経痛」と診断され、針灸治療を求めた。

検査：Lasegue's の徴候（+）。舌苔が白く、脈は弦であった。

診断：痺症（坐骨神経痛）。

治療経過：環跳、陽陵泉、足三里、崑崙などの穴を取り（環跳穴には、0.85％NaClを20ml 1回注射する）、治療後、痛みがただちに止まり、立って歩くことができた。7回の治療で治癒した。

例7： 针刺治疗心绞痛，止痛迅速。

陈××，女，37岁，住院号204849。

主诉：前胸疼痛，已1年余。

现病史：1年前，无诱因而感前胸发作性灼痛，向左肩放散，夜间发作明显，一夜达2～4次，1次持续数分钟。每遇过劳、精神紧张时发作加剧。入院后服西药无效，而请中医会诊。

舌脉：舌隐青，苔白，脉弦。

诊断：胸痹（心绞痛）。

治疗经过：取膻中、内关（双），留针20分钟，针后5分钟疼痛即止。为巩固疗效又针治2次后基本控制，病人出院。

Example 7: Acupuncture treatment of angina pectoris with rapid relief of pain.

Chen ××, Female, Age 37, Case No 204849.

Chief Complaint: Pain in the anterior chest for more than a year.

History of Illness: There was a paroxysmal burning pain in the anterior chest without any apparent reason. The pain radiated to right shoulder. The onset was evident during the night, and the pain occurred 2～4 times a night. Each attack of pain lasted for several minuts. The attacks were worsened by overwork or tension. After admission she had been treatment with western medicine which was found ineffective. Consultation by doctors practising traditional Chinese medicine was requested.

Tongue and Pulse: Purplish tongue with white coat and wiry

pulse.

Diagnosis: Chest Bi(Stenocardia).

Treatment: Shanzhong, Neiguan (on both sides) were given with retention of the needles for 20 minutes. Pain was relieved five minutes after acupuncture. The condition was generally controlled with another two acupuncture treatments. The patient was then discharged.

例7: 狭心症は、針刺で痛みがすみやかに止まる。

陳××、女、37才、住院番号204879。

主訴：前胸部に痛みがあって1年余り。

現病歴：1年前から、特に誘因もなく、前胸部に発作性のしゃく痛を感じ、左肩部に放射する。とくに夜間発作が明らかで、1夜に2～4回発作を起し、1回は数分間持続する。過労あるいは精神的に緊張した時に発作が激しくなる。入院後は、西洋薬を内服したが、あまり効果がなく、漢方治療を求めた。

舌脈：舌はやや青く、舌苔は白く、脈は弦であった。

診断：胸痺（狭心症）。

治療経過：膻中、内関（両側）に刺し、20分間留針する。治療後5分間で、痛みが止まる。効果を持続させるため、さらに2回針刺して、症状消失したため退院した。

例8: 针刺10次，痹证治愈。

焦××，男，59岁。

主诉：膝关节疼痛已1年。

现病史：1年前，劳累后发现两膝关节酸痛，但局部不红、不肿，阴雨天疼痛加剧。曾服中、西药治疗，效果不理想，要求针灸治疗。

舌脉：舌红，苔黄厚，脉弦。

诊断：痹证（两膝关节痛）。

治疗经过，取鹤顶、犊鼻、内膝眼、足三里等穴，每日1次，1次20分钟。第1次治疗后即感两腿轻松，疼痛减轻。针10次后治愈。

Example 8: Bi syndrome cured with ten acupuncture treatments.

Jiao ××, Male, Age 59.

Chief Complaint: Arthralgia of both knees for one year.

History of Illness: Both knees suffered from arthralgia after over use for one year but without local redness and swelling. The pain became severe during overcast and rainy days. The patient was given traditional Chinese medicines and western medicines. The results were not satisfactory, so the patient came for acupuncture treatment.

Tongue and Pulse: Red tongue with thick yellow coating, and wiry pulse.

Diagnosis: Bi syndrome (Arthralgia of both knees).

Treatment: Selected points of Heding, Dubi, Internal Xiyan, Zusanli, etc. once for 20 minuts a day. The patient felt that both legs were lighter and easier and more comfortable with less pain after the first treatment. The patient's condition was improved with ten acupuncture treatments.

例8： 針刺10回で、痺症治癒。

焦××、男、59才。

主訴：両側の膝関節の痛みに苦しんで1年。

現病歴： 1年前に過労した後、両膝関節がだるくて痛み、局所には、発赤や腫れはない、曇った日や雨の日などは特に痛みがひどくなる。漢方薬と西洋薬を服用したが、効果が理想的でないため、針灸治療を求めた。

舌脈：舌が赤く、舌苔は黄色で厚く、脈は弦でした。

診断：痺症（両膝関節痛）。

治療経過：鶴頂、犢鼻、内膝眼、足三里などの穴を取り、1日1回の治療で、毎回20分間留針する。第1回の治療で、両足が楽になり、痛みも軽減した。10回で、治癒した。

例9： 針刺20次，使听力恢复正常。

王××，男，21岁，住院号227469。

主诉：患流脑后并发失明，耳聋，尿潴留。

现病史：患"流脑"入传染科治疗已3天。因伴有失明、耳聋、尿潴

留，而请针灸科会诊。

舌脉：舌质红、苔黄、脉弦数。

诊断：流脑并发失明、耳聋、尿潴留。

治疗经过：取穴上廉泉、外金津、玉液、中极、横骨、三阴交、耳门、听宫、翳风、外关。

第1次针治后能自动排尿，可发音说1个字，治疗5次后能说话，听力有所恢复，拍手时有反应。治疗20次后听力恢复正常。

Example 9: Hearing returned to normal with twenty acupuncture treatments.

Wang ××, Male, Age 21, Case No 227469.

Chief Complaint: After having suffered epidemic cerebrospinal meningitis, the patient's condition was complicated by blindness, deafness, and urinary retention.

History of Illness: Three days previously, the patient had been admitted to the infectious diseases department because of blindness, deafness and urinary retention, requesting consultation for acupuncture and moxibustion treatment.

Tongue and Pulse: Red, yellow-coated tongue, wiry and rapid pulse.

Diagnosis: Epidemic cerebrospinal meningitis complicated by blindness, deafness and urinary retention.

Treatment: Selected Upper Lianquan, External Jinjn, Yuye, Zhongji, Henggu, Sanyinjiao, Ermen, Tinggong, Yifeng, Waiguan.

The patient could pass water voluntarily and state one word after the first acupuncture treatment. With five acupuncture treatments the patient was able to speak, and respond to clapping hands showing that hearing was recovering to some extent. After twenty acupuncture treatments hearing became normal.

例9：針刺20回で、聴力が正常に回復。

王××、男、21才、住院番号227469。

主訴：流行性髄膜炎に罹って、失明、難聴、尿閉を併発した。

現病歷：患者は流行性髄膜炎で傳染科に入院して3日目。失明、難

聴と尿閉を併発しているので、針灸科に対診を求めた。
　舌脈：舌質が赤く、舌苔は黄色、脈は弦数であった。
　診断：流行性髄膜炎合併失明、難聴、尿閉。
　治療経過：上廉泉、外金津、玉液、中極、横骨、三陰交、耳門、聴宮、翳風、外関などの穴を取った。1回の治療で自主排尿と一つの音節を発することができ、5回の治療後には話すことができ、聴力の回復もみられ、拍手する時に反応がある。20回の治療で聴力が正常に回復した。

　例10：针刺治疗月经过多。
　刘××，女，36岁，住院号209448。
　主诉：月经量多不止。
　现病史：患者因眼病在眼科住院行眼手术，术后为经期第1天，因月经量多不止，而请针灸科会诊。
　舌脉：舌淡、苔白、脉弦。
　诊断：月经过多。
　治疗经过：取中极、血海、三阴交等穴，首次针后，血量明显减少，2次针治后即恢复正常。

Example 10: Treatment of menorrhagia by acupuncture
Liu ××, Female, Age 36, Case No 209448.
Chief Complaint: Menorrhagia.
History of illness: The patient was admitted to the ophthalmology department for an eye operation. After operation, on the first day of menstruation, the quantity of blood was excessive and persistent. Consultation for acupuncture and moxibustion was requested.
Tongue and Pulse: Pale, white-coated tongue, wiry pulse.
Diagnosis: Excessive menstruation.
Treatment: Selected points of Zhongji, Xuehai, Sanyinjiao, etc. The quantity of blood decreased markedly after the first acupuncture treatment and the condition became normal after two acupuncture treatments.

例10：月経過多の針刺治療。

劉××、女、36才、住院番号209448。

主訴：月経の量が多くて止まらない。

現病歴：患者は目の病気で眼科に入院して、目の手術を受きたもので、術後月経の1日目に月経の量が多く、止まらないため、針灸治療を求めた。

舌脈：舌がうすく、舌苔は白く、脈は弦であった。

診断：月経過多。

治療経過：中極、血海、三陰交などの穴を取り、1回刺した後、量が明らかに減り、2回で正常に回復した。

例11：针刺治疗重症肌无力，疗效明显。

刘××，女，16岁，住院号228348。

主诉：四肢及全身肌肉无力已1年余。

现病史：患者1年来无诱因而感四肢及全身肌肉无力，并逐渐加重。1985年3月10日入神经科住院。入院20余日，用药物治疗，效果欠佳，而要求针灸治疗。

查体：患者卧位，不能翻身、抬头和抬高四肢，张口困难仅一横指，舌胖，苔白，脉弦。

诊断：重症肌无力。

治疗经过：

取穴：地仓，颊车、下关、夹脊穴（胸6、7，腰2、3），环跳、秩边、足三里、承山、昆仑、肩髃、曲池、外关、合谷。

针治1次张口至二横指，四肢可抬高、翻身，3次后能坐起，5次后即可站立，10次后可迈步。共治疗2个月，恢复到可做一般活动。1986年及1987年随访2年，疗效巩固。

Example 11: Myasthenia gvavis showed mraked improvement with acupuncture treatment.

Liu ××, Female, Age 16, Case No 228348.

Chief Complaint: The body showed generalized myasthenia for over a year, particularly the extremeties.

History of Illness: For a year the patient has felt myasthenia in the extremities and all over the body with no apparent cause. The condition has become gradually more severe. The patient was admitted to the neurology department on March 10, 1985, and was given drugs for more than twenty days. The result was not satisfactorily effective. The consultation for acupuncture and moxibustion was requested.

Physical Examination: The patient was in a position of decubitus and could not turn her body, raise her head, or elevate her extremities. There was difficulty in opening her mouth, she could only open to the extent of one finger-breadth. The tongue was swollen and white coated and the pulse was wiry.

Diagnosis: Myasthenia gravis.

Treatment: Selected points of Dicang, Jiache, Xiaguan, Jiaji (Chest 6,7, lumbar 2,3), Huantiao, Zhibian, Zusanli, Chengshan, kunlun, Jianju, Quchi, Waiguan, Hegu.

The patient's mouth opened to two finger breadths wide, the extremities could be raised high and she could turn her body after the first treatment. The patient could sat up after three treatments and could stand after five treatments. She was able to take a step after ten treatments. The patient returned to her general activities after two months' treatment. Follow-up visits in 1986 and 1987 showed steady theraputic effect.

例11：重症の筋無力症、針刺治療で、効果顕著。

劉××、女、16才、住院番号228348。

主訴：四肢及び全身筋肉無力で1年あまり。

現病歴：患者は1年以来、何らの誘因なく、四肢と全身の筋肉無力を感じ、次第に重くなり、1985年3月10日に神経科に住院した。20日間の薬物治療で、余り改善されず、針灸治療を希望した。

検査：患者は臥位で、寝返りができない。頭をあげるのと四肢を上挙することもできなく、口は1横指しかあけられず、舌が肥大し、舌苔は白く、脈は弦である。

診断：重症の筋無力症。

治療経過：

取穴：地倉、頬車、下関、夾脊穴（胸6、7と腰2、3）、環跳、秩辺、足三里、承山、崑崙、肩髃、曲池、外関、合谷。

1回の治療で、口が2横指まであけられ、四肢の上挙と寝返りができた。5回で立つことが出来、10回で歩行可能となった。2ケ月の治療で、普通の活動が出来るように回復した。1986年と1987年の訪問で、治療効果は持続していた。

例12：针刺治疗一氧化碳中毒后遗症。

马××，女，45岁，住院号227656。

主诉：神志呆滞已10余天。

现病史：患者于1个月前煤气中毒，当时昏迷48小时，醒后无异常；20天后出现发呆，少话，傻笑，计算力差，二便无知觉等症状，2月25日到神经科住院，治疗效果欠佳，而请针灸科会诊。

舌脉：舌胖，苔薄白，脉弦。

诊断：一氧化碳中毒后遗症。

治疗经过：取百会、四神聪、神门、内关、太冲、中极、横骨、三阴交等穴。

针治2次后出现排尿、排便感，针治4次后计算力有改善，20次后神志恢复如常，能正确对话。

Example 12: Acupuncture treatment for delayed effects of carbon monoxide poisoning.

Ma××, Female, Age 45, Case No 227656.

Chief Complaint: Dull appearance for more than ten days.

History of Illness: The patient suffered gas poisoning one month previously and was comatose for 48 hours at that time without any abnormality after waking up. Trance-like symptoms occurred, with lack of speech, foolish laughter, poor calculation ability and urinary and faecal incontinence twenty days later. The patient was admitted to the neurology department on February 25. The result of treatment was not satisfactory so the acupuncture and moxibustion was accepted.

Tongue and pulse: Swollen, thinly white-coated tongue, wiry pulse.

Diagnosis: Delayed effects of carbon monoxide poisoning.
Treatment: Baihui, Sishencong, Shenmen, Neiguan, Taichong, Zhongji, Henggu, Sanyinjiao, etc. were selected. Awareness of urination and defecation occurred after two acupuncture treatments. The ability to calculate improved after four acupuncture treatments, mental condition returned to normal, and the patient could talk with others normally after twenty acupuncture treatments.

例12：一酸化炭素中毒の後遺症を針刺で治療。
馬××、女、45才、住院号227656。
主訴：神志がぼんやりして10日あまり。
現病歴：患者は1个月前にガス中毒のため、48時間昏迷した。さめた後は異常なかったが、20日後から神志がぼんやりして、口数も少なくなり、げらげら笑うばかりで、計算する能力が減退し、大便と小便の感覚がないなどの症状が現われた。2月25日に神経科に入院したが、効果がよくないため、針灸科の対診を求めた。
舌脈：舌が肥大し、舌苔はうす白く、脈は弦であった。
診断：一酸化炭素中毒後遺症。
治療経過：百会、四神聡、神門、内関、太衝、中極、横骨、三陰交などの穴を取り、針治療2回で、排尿と排便の感じが出てきた。4回の治療で計算能力がよくなり、20回で神志が正常に回復し、正確に対話することができるようになった。

例13：流脑并发失语、偏瘫验例。
高××，女，22岁，住院号226440。
主诉：失语、右半身瘫已10余天。
现病史：病人因高热，头痛，被诊断为"流脑"入传染科住院治疗后症状有好转，但失语和右半身瘫10余日来不见好转，故请会诊。
舌脉：舌质红，苔薄黄，脉弦。
诊断：流脑并发失语、偏瘫。
治疗经过：
　　取穴：外金津、玉液，
　　　　　右侧曲池、外关、手三里、合谷、阳陵泉、足三里、丰隆、

昆仑。

针治1次后，可发单音，右下肢可稍活动。6次后能说话，上、下肢均可活动。20次后行走如常。

Example 13: An example of successful acupuncture treatment of epidemic cerebrospinal meningitis complicated by aphasia and hemiplegia.

Gao ××, Female, Age 22, Case No 226440.

Chief Complaint: Aphasia, right-sided hemiplegia for more than ten days.

History of Illness: The patient was diagnosed as "epidemic cerebrospinal meningitis" because of high fever and headache. The patient was therefore admitted to the infectious diseases department. The symptoms showed improvement but aphasia and hemiplegia of the right side persisted. Consultation for acupuncture treatment was requested.

Tongue and Pulse: Red, thinly yellow-coated tongue; wiry pulse.

Diagnosis: Epidemic cerebrospinal meningitis complicated by aphasia, hemiplegia.

Treatment:

Selected points: External Jinjin, Yuji, and Quchi, Waiguan, Shousanli, Hegu, Yanglingquan, Zusanli, Fenglong, kunlun on the right side.

The patient could pronounce single phonations, the right-lower extremity could react slightly after the first acupuncture treatment. The patient could speak. The upper and lower extremities could move after six acupuncture treatments and she could walk as usuual after twenty acupuncture treatments.

例13：流行性髄膜炎の失語と半身不遂を合併した症例。

高××、女、22才、住院番号226440。

主訴：失語と右半身不遂で10日あまり。

現病歴：患者は高熱、頭痛があり、流行性髄膜炎と診断され、伝染

科に入院し、治療により症状が改善されたが、失語と右半身不遂は、10日あまりになっても、なおよくならず、対診を求めた。

舌脈：舌質が赤く、舌苔はうすく黄色。脈は弦であった。

診断：流行性髄膜炎合併失語、半身不遂。

治療経過：

　取穴：外金津、玉液。

　　　右側曲池、外関、手三里、合谷、陽陵泉、足三里、豊隆、崑崙。

1回で、単音を発することができ、右下肢が少し動けるようになり、6回の治療で会話及び上肢と下肢もみな活動することができるようになった。20回で正常に歩行できるようになった。

例14：针刺8次，眼肌麻痹治愈。

韩××，男，28岁，住院号227671。

主诉：右眼睑下垂，不能上提已2个月。

现病史：患者3个月前无诱因而发右头部剧痛，2个月前又出现右眼睑下垂，不能上抬。用激素治疗曾一度好转，现仍有右眼睑下垂，并出现复视，而请针灸科会诊。

舌脉：舌质红，苔薄黄，脉弦。

诊断：疼痛性眼肌麻痹。

治疗经过：取右侧睛明、攒竹、太阳、阳白透鱼腰、风池、合谷等穴。

针治1次右眼睑即可上提，视物双影间距缩小，8次后痊愈。

Example 14: Ophthalmoplegia cured with eight acupuncture treatments.

Han ××, Male, Age 28, Case No 227671.

Chief Complaint: Ptosis of the right eyelid could not be raised for two months.

History of Illness: Three months previously, the patient had developed a severe headache on the right side with no apparent cause. Ptosis of the right eyelid occurred one month later and the right eyelid could not be raised. The condition improved following hormone treatment. However, ptosis of the right eyelid re-occurred and double vision developed. The acupuncncture and moxibustion treatment then started.

Tongue and Pulse: Red tongue, with a thin yellow coating; wiry pulse.

Diagnosis: Painful ophthalmoplegia.

Treatment: Selected Jingming, Zanzhu, Taiyang, penetration of Yangbai towards Yuyao, Fengchi, Hegu, etc. on the right.

The right eyelid could be raised after one acupuncture treatment. The distance between the double vision images was reduced, and then completely cured after eight treatments.

例14：眼筋麻痺が、針治療8回で治癒。

韓××、男、28才、住院番号227671。

主訴：右眼瞼が下垂して、上げることが出来ないようになって2个月。

現病歷：患者は3个月前、何ら誘因がなく、右頭部が激しく痛み、2个月前から右眼瞼が下垂し、あげることができなくなり、ホルモン剤で治療の結果一度よくなり、今は、なお右眼瞼下垂があり、同時に複視が現われて、針灸科の対診を要求した。

舌脈：舌質が赤く、舌苔は薄黄、脈は弦であった。

診断：疼痛性眼筋麻痺。

治療経過：右側睛明、攢竹、太陽、陽白と魚腰を透刺し、風池、合谷などの穴を取った。1回の治療で右眼瞼をあげることができ、物を見る時、二重影の距離が小さくなり、8回で完全に治癒した。

例15：针刺治疗带状疱疹效果显著。

李××，男，43岁，门诊号8653。

主诉：右颈背部剧痛已1周。

现病史：患者于1周前，突感右颈背部剧痛，继而出现小丘疹水疱，5～6个聚集成堆。经皮肤科诊为"带状疱疹"。服用激素类药物未见效，痛剧不能入睡，而来要求针灸治疗。

舌脉：舌体胖，苔薄黄，脉弦。

诊断：带状疱疹。

治疗经过：取风池、太冲和局部阿是穴。针治1次后，疼痛减轻而能入睡，5次后完全治愈。

Example 15: Outstanding therapeutic effect on herpes zoster with acupuncture treatment.

Li ××, Male, Age 43, Chart No 8653.

Chief Complaint: Sharp pain to the back and right of the neck for one week.

History of Illness: The patient felt sudden severe pain to the back part of the right side of the neck. Then after a short time blistering occurred. Five or six blisters were grouped. "Herpes zoster" was diagnosed by the dermatologist. The patient was given hormone treatment without effect. He could not sleep because of the sharp pain. Acupuncture treatment started then.

Tongue and Pulse: The body of the tongue was swollen, the tongue was thinly yellow-coated, wiry pulse.

Diagnosis: Herpes zoster.

Treatment: Selected Fengchi, Taichong, and local Ashi points. The pain was relieved and the patient was able to sleep after only one acupuncture treatment. The patient recovered completely after five acupuncture treatments.

例15：針治療は帯状疱疹に顕著な効果がある。

李××、男、43才、外来8653。

主訴：右頸背部激しく痛んで1週間になる。

現病歴：患者は、1週間前に突然右頸背部に激しい痛みが現われ、つづいて小さい丘疹様水疱が出た。5～6個集まって積みかさね、帯状疱疹と皮膚科で診断をつけられ、ホルモン剤で効果なく、痛みが激しくねむれないので、針灸治療に外来した。

舌脈：舌体が肥大し、舌苔はうすく黄色、脈は弦。

診断：帯状疱疹。

治療経過：風池、太衝と局所の阿是穴を取り、1回の治療で、痛みが軽減し寝むれるようになり、5回で完全に治癒した。

第七章 耳针疗法

耳针疗法，是指用针刺等方法刺激耳穴以防治疾病的一种方法。耳针疗法早在《黄帝内经》一书中就有记载，几千年来一直为我国人民所应用，近年来，在继承发扬祖国医学的同时，还参考国外有关资料，进行了广泛的研究，使其更加丰富。下面就这一疗法，作简要介绍。

Chapter Ⅶ Ear Acupuncture Therapy

Ear acupuncture therapy treats diseases by stimulating certain points of the auricle with needles. Such a method of treatment was recorded as early as in the book Neijing(500-300B.C.).This therapeutic method has long been used by the people of china for thousands of years. Our medical workers have inherited and promoted traditional Chinese medicine, while also studying foreign texts in order to make a comprehensive study of ear acupuncture. It has greatly broadened the realm of ear acupuncture therapy in recent years. The technique is briefly described as follows:

第七章 耳針療法

耳針療法とは、耳介にある穴に針刺などの方法を施して、疾病を預防し、治療する方法をいう。耳針療法は「黄帝内経」に早くから記載されていた。数千年の長期にわたって、人民に応用されてきた。ここ数年来、中国の医務関係者は、祖国の医学をうけつぎ、発掘すると同時に、外国の耳針療法に関する資料を参照して、幅広く研究を進めた。したがって、耳針療法の内容はもとの基礎のうえで更に豊富になった。次にこの治療法について簡単に紹介する。

第一节 耳与经络、脏腑的关系

中医认为：耳不是一个孤立的器官，耳廓与经络、脏腑有着密切的联系，它和全身是一个统一的有机整体。《内经》中指出，十二经脉，三百六十五络，它们的气血都上行于面，并走于耳，使耳听觉功能正常。如手太阳、手阳明和手、足少阳四经均入耳，足阳明和足太阳经脉联系到耳的周围，即六条阳经皆到耳。而六条阴经也通过其支脉与耳部有联系。奇经八脉也入耳。故耳部有许多经脉聚会。

耳与脏腑：肾开窍于耳。肾气足可使听力正常。如肾虚（老年人则肾虚）精少，可出现耳鸣耳聋等。正常情况下，人体各部之间的生理功能保持相对的平衡和协调。一旦失去平衡，经络阻滞，在耳廓上的相应部位就可出现反应。临床上针刺耳穴，以疏通经络，运行气血，调整脏腑，就能治疗全身各部的有关病证。

I. Relations between the Auricle and Channels, Collaterals and Zang-Fu Organs

It is held in traditional Chinese medicine that the ear is not a separate organ but closely connected with channels and collaterals and zang-fu organs, and is a part of the body as an organic whole. As is pointed out in Neijing, the qi and blood of all twelve channels and their 365 collaterals ascend to the face reaching the ear to make auditory function normal. For instance, the Small Intestine Channel of Hand-Taiyang, Large Intestine Channel of Hand-Yangming, Sanjiao Channel of Hand-Shaoyang and Gallbladder Channel of Foot-Shaoyang enter the ear, while the Stomach Channel of Foot-Yangming and Urinary Bladder Channel of Foot-Taiyang reach the periauricular region. The six yang channels all enter the ear while the six yin channels connect with the ear through the branches of the channels. The eight extra channels enter the ear. Therefore the ear is the converging site of a number of channels.

The ear and zang-fu organs: The kidney is opening into the ear. Ample storage of the qi of the kidney makes the auditory function of the ear normal. For instance, insufficiency of essence in the kidney may give rise to tinnitus and deafness, and so on. (Old people may have poor kidney function.) In normal conditions, a relative balance and co-ordination is maintained among the physiological functions of the various parts of the body. Once an imbalance and incoordination are present and channel stasis occurs, reactions can be detected at the corresponding areas on the auricle. Clinically, diseases of various parts of the body can be cured by needling the corresponding auricular points, which may promote free circulation of qi and blood in the channels and collaterals and adjust the zang-fu organs.

第一節　耳と経絡・臓腑との関係

　　中医学では、耳は一つの孤立した器官ではなくて、耳介と経絡・臓腑とは密接につながっており、全身を一つの統一的な有機的な生体として考える。「内経」には、「十二経脈と三百六十五絡脈の気血は、すべて顔面と脳髄に上行し、その中の別行された気血が耳に行って、耳の聴覚を正常にさせる」と指摘している。例えば、手太陽経、手陽明経と手・足少陽経の4本の経脈は耳中に入り、足陽明経と足太陽経が耳の周囲に分布する。即ち、六本の陽経の経脈がそれぞれ耳の中と耳の周囲に行き、六本の陰経は、直接は耳に入らないが、その支脈により耳とつながっている。奇経八脈も耳に入り、したがって、耳には数多くの経脈が集中されていることになる。

　　耳と臓腑との関係については、腎は耳に開竅し、腎気が旺盛であれば、聴覚を正常にし、腎虚精少（老年になると腎虚になる）になると、耳鳴、難聴などが現われてくる。正常な状態では、人体各部の生理機能は、相対的なバランスと協調を保つことができるが、一旦このバランス関係がくずれると、経脈が滞り、耳介にある対応部位に反応が出現してくる。臨床においては、耳穴を針刺して、経絡を疏通させ、気血の運行をととのえ、臓腑の働きを調節することにより、全身各部の疾患を治療

することができる。

第二节 耳针的穴位

耳穴是指耳廓上的一些特定的刺激点。当人体内脏或躯体有病时，往往会在耳廓的一定部位出现各种反应，如压痛敏感、皮肤电阻变低、变形、变色等。医者可以利用这些现象作为诊断疾病时的参考。并可刺激这些部位以防治疾病。

耳穴的分布规律：可概括为"一个倒立的人"，如：头面部相应的穴位在耳垂；上肢相应的穴位在耳舟；躯干和下肢相应的穴位在对耳轮和对耳轮上、下脚；内脏相应的穴位在耳甲艇和耳甲腔（图63）。

II. Auricular Points

Auricular points are specific points to which stimuli are given for treatment of disease. When disorders occur in the internal organs or other parts of the body, various reactions may appear at the corresponding parts of the auricle, such as tenderness, decreased resistance to electric current, morphological changes and discoloration. In making a diagnosis, these phenomena can be taken into consideration. Application of stimuli to the sensitive sites serves to prevent and treat disease.

Distribution of auricular points: This may be summarized as "a person standing on his head." Such as points that are located at the lobule are related to the head and facial region, those on the scapha to the upper limbs, those on the antihelix and its two crura to the trunk and lower limbs, and those in the cavum and cymba conchae to the internal organs (Fig 63).

第二節　耳針の穴位

　　耳穴とは、耳介にある特定の刺激点を指す。人体の内臓および体が罹患した時、往々にして耳介のある部位にいろいろな反応が現われてくる。例えば、圧痛敏感、皮膚の電気抵抗低下、変形、変色などのような現象である。医者は、これを診断の参考とする。そして、これらの部位に刺激を与えることにより疾病を治療することができる。

　　耳穴分布は、「さかたちした人」と似ている。一般には、頭部顔面部に相応する穴位は耳垂にあり、上肢に相応する穴位は舟状窩に分布し、軀幹と下肢に相応する穴位は対輪脚、上対輪脚と下対輪脚にあり、内臓に相応する穴位は多く耳甲介艇と耳甲介腔に分布する（図63）。

第三节　耳针的临床应用

选穴原则

　　根据病变部位选穴，即根据病变部位在耳廓上选取相应的耳穴。如胃痛选胃穴，肩痛选肩穴。

　　根据脏腑、经络学说选穴，即根据脏腑的生理、经络循行以及其表里关系为依据，选取有关耳穴。如肺主皮毛，故皮肤病可选肺穴。心与小肠相表里，心悸可选小肠穴。头颞部与少阳胆经有关，故偏头痛可选胆穴。

　　根据现代医学知识选穴，即要以现代生理、病理为指导，选

有关耳穴。如月经不调选内分泌穴,腹痛选交感穴。

也有根据主要症状,随症选穴治疗。如耳赤肿痛选耳尖,咽喉肿痛选用轮1~6。

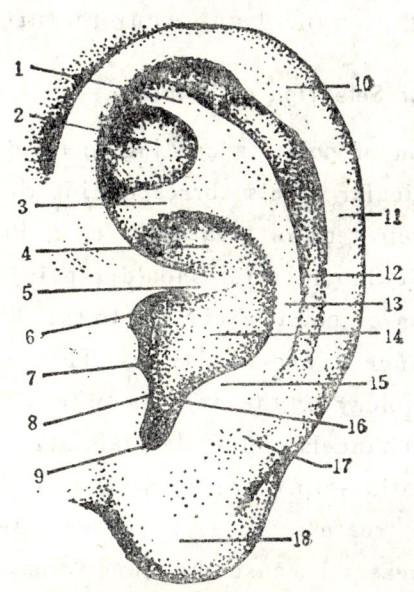

图(Fig)63 耳廓表面解剖名称
(Anatomy of the surface of the auricle)
1. 对耳轮上脚 (Superior antihelix crus)
2. 三角窝 (Triangular fossa)
3. 对耳轮下脚 (Inferior antihelix crus)
4. 耳甲艇 (Cymba conchae)
5. 耳轮脚 (Helix crus)
6. 屏上切迹 (Supratragic notch)
7. 外耳道口 (Orifice of external auditory meatus)
8. 耳　屏 (Tragus)
9. 屏间切迹 (Intertragic notch)
10. 耳轮结节 (Auricular tubercle)
11. 耳　轮 (Helix)
12. 耳　舟 (Scapha)
13. 对耳轮 (Antihelix)
14. 耳甲腔 (Cavum conchae)
15. 屏轮切迹 (Notch between antitragus and antihelix)
16. 对耳屏 (Antitragus)
17. 耳轮屏 (Helix cauda)
18. 耳　垂 (Lobule)

III. Clinical Application of Ear Acupuncture

Rules for Selection of Points

Selection of points according to the diseased areas. That is, auricular points corresponding to the diseased areas are selected for treatment, e.g. Pt. Stomach for gastralgia, Pt. Shoulder for shoulder pain.

Selection of points according to the theories of zang-fu and channels and collaterals. That is, on the basis of the physiology of the zang-fu organs, courses of circulation of channels and collaterals and their external-internal relationship, corresponding auricular points are selected for treatment. E.g., Pt. Lung can be selected for skin diseases because the lung dominates the skin and hair; Pt. Small Intestine for palpitation as the heart is externally-internally related to the small intestine; Pt. Gall bladder for temporal headache as the temporal region is supplied by the Gall bladder Channel of Foot-Shaoyang.

Selection of points in terms of modern medicine. That is, auricular points are selected with physiological and pathological consideration, e.g. Pt. Endocrine is selected for irregular menstruation, Pt. Sympathetic Nerve for abdominal pain.

In addition, auricular points can be selected according to the cardinal symptoms of a disease, e.g. Pt.

Ear Apex for redness, swelling and pain of the eye, Pts.Helix 1〜6 for sore throat.

第三節　耳針の臨床応用

選穴原則

　病変の部位による取穴：即ち病気の部位によって、耳介上に相応の穴を選ぶ。例えば、胃痛は胃穴を取り、肩痛には肩穴を取る。

　臓腑経絡学説による取穴：即ち、臓腑の生理、経絡循行および表裏関係を根拠にして、関係ある耳穴を取る。「肺は皮毛を主る」という理論により、皮膚病の場合、よく肺穴を取る。心と小腸が表裏関係にあるので、心悸には小腸穴を取ってもよい。側頭部は足少陽胆経と関連あるから、側頭痛にはよく胆穴を選ぶ。

　現代医学知識による取穴：これは、主に現代生理病理学の指導のもとに関連ある穴を取る。例えば、月経不順には内分泌穴を選ぶ。腹痛には交感穴を選ぶ。

　このほか、疾病の主な症状により、耳穴を取る。例えば、目赤腫痛の場合、耳尖を選び、咽喉腫痛には、輪1〜6を選ぶ。

操作方法

　寻找反应点：在选用的穴区寻找反应点，其方法有二，一是压痛探查法，用探针在相应部位由周围向中心探压，找明显压痛点，稍加压力，作为针刺记号。二是电探测法，是采用一定的仪器测定耳穴的电阻、电容、电位等变化。

　消毒：用75％酒精或2％碘酒在耳穴消毒。

　进针：左手固定耳廓，右手持0.5寸或1寸毫针对准穴位快速

刺入，深度以不透过对侧皮肤为度。针刺时一般较痛，有时会出现热、胀、酸、重等感觉，有以上反应者疗效较好。

留针：一般留针20～30分钟，对某些急性炎症，痛证和发作性疾病也可留针1～2小时或更长些。在留针期间可间歇性给以运针手法。

出针：拔针后以消毒干棉球压迫针孔，以防出血。

疗程：每天或隔日1次，10次为1疗程，疗程间可休3～7天。

Techniques of Ear Acupuncture

Probing of the sensitive spot: There are two common methods of probing for the sensitive spots at the areas where the selected points are located.(a) One is probing for the tender spot. Probe with a blunt needle around the selected point on the auricle from the rim towards the centre. When marked tenderness is located, press hard to mark the spot for applying acupuncture. (b) The other is probing by electric apparatus. That is to observe the changes in electric resistance, capacity and potential at the areas of the selected auricular points with a special apparatus.

Aseptic procedure: Auricular points are swabbed with 75% alcohol or 2% iodine.

Insertion of needle: Stabilize the auricle with the left hand. Hold a filiform needle of 0.5 or 1 cun with the right hand and insert it swiftly into the point avoiding penetration of the ear. There is generally a sensation of pain, but sometimes of hotness, distension, soreness or heaviness, any of which usually signify satisfactory therapeutic result.

Retention of needle: Needles are usually retained for 20~30 minutes, but in acute inflammatory cases, severe pain and paroxysmal seizures, needles are retained for 1~2 hours or even longer and intermittently manipulated to enhance stimulation.

Removal of needle: After the needle is removed, press the puncture hole with a dry, sterile cotton ball to avoid infection.

Course of treatment: Treatment is given once every day or every other day. Ten treatments make a course. The interval between courses is 3~7 days.

操作方法

反応点を捜す：選ばれた穴位区に反応点を捜す。常用する探査方法は二つある。その一つは圧痛探査法で、プローバで耳介の相応部位で周囲から中心にむかって、圧を加えながら探査を行い、著明な圧痛点をさがしだす。そして、その部に軽く少し圧を加えると、くぼみが出来るから、その出来たくぼみを目印とする。もう一つの方法は、電気抵抗探査法で、一定の測定器で耳穴の電気抵抗、電気容量、電位などの変化を測る方法である。

消毒：75％のアルコールあるいは2％のヨードチンキで耳穴を消毒する。

進針：左手で耳介を固定し、右手で0.5寸或は1寸の毫針を持って、正確にすばやく耳穴に刺し、刺入の深さは、反対側の皮膚を穿透しない程度がよい。針刺する時、一般にはかなり痛みがあり、場合によっては、熱い、はれぼったい、だるい、重たいなどの感じがある。

置針：普通は20～30分間置針する。急性炎症あるいは痛症

と発作性疾患には1〜2時間、場合によっては更に長く置針することもある。置針中には間歇的に捻針して、刺激を強める。

抜針：出血を防ぐため抜針してから消毒乾棉球で押える。

クール：一般には、毎日あるいは隔日に1回治療し、10回を1クールとする。次のクールとの間隔は3〜7日である。

注意事項

同针灸的一般注意事项。

如留针过程中，在病变无关的其他部位突然发生疼痛、酸、胀等，可将针后退或拔出反应可消失。

对扭伤及肢体活动障碍的病人，进针后待耳廓充血发热时，宜嘱病人适当活动肢体对患部按摩，加灸有助于疗效的提高。

Remarks

The remarks here are similar to the general remarks applying to acupuncture and moxibustion.

Such as, if sudden pain, soreness or distension occurs with retained needle at an area not within that of the disease being treated, it is advisable to lift the needle a little or remove it so that the abnormal feeling disappears.

In treating a patient with sprain or motor impairment of the extremities, it is necessary after the needle has produced heat from congestion in the auricle to ask the patient to move the affected limb, or apply massage or moxibustion to the affected part in order to enhance the therapeutic effect.

注意事項

注意すべきことは、普通の針灸療法の注意事項と同じである。

もし、置針中、疾病と無関係の部位に、疼痛、だるい、はれぼったいなどの不快感がある時は、針をやや浅くするか、全部取り出せば、消失させることが出来る。

捻挫傷及び肢体運動障害の患者には、針を刺しいれて耳介に発熱充血の感じが生じた場合、患者に適当に肢体を運かさせるか、患部を按摩して、お灸を施せば、治療効果は一層高められる。

常见病症的耳针选穴举例（图64）

头痛——皮质下、额、枕或太阳。
失眠——神门、心、枕或额、皮质下。
呃逆——膈。
哮喘——平喘、肺、肾上腺。
急性扭挫伤——相应部位耳穴、皮质下、神门。
痛经——子宫、内分泌、肝。
急性结膜炎——眼、肝或耳尖。
听力减退——内耳、肾。
荨麻疹——肺、肝、脾。

Examples of Selection of Points for Common Diseases (Fig. 64)

Headache: Subcortex, Forehead, Occiput or Taiyang.

Insomnia: Ear-Shenmen, Heart, Forehead or Occiput, Subcortex.

Hiccup: Diaphragm.

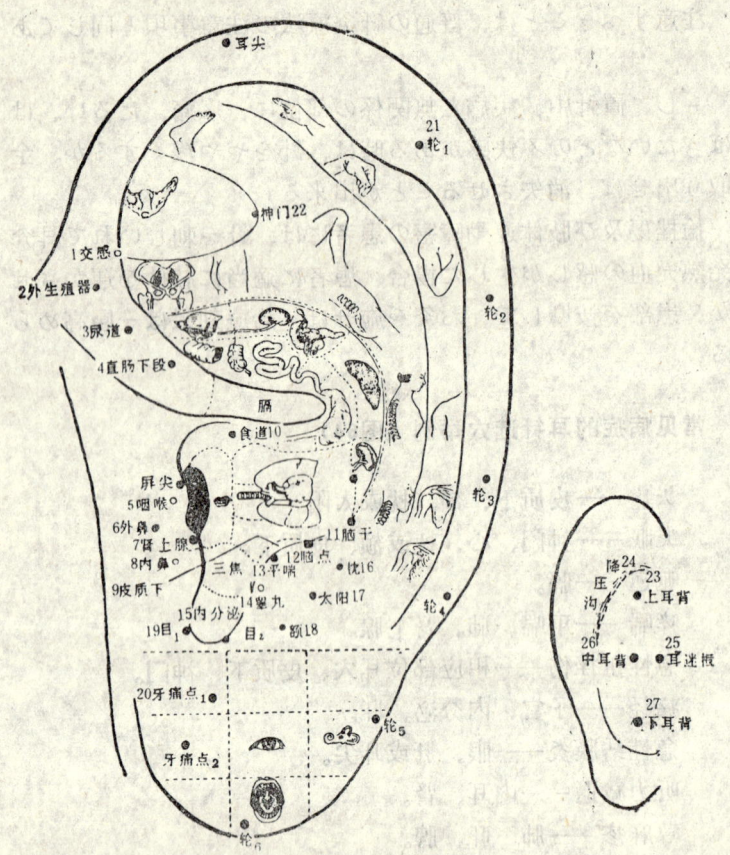

图(Fig.)64 常用耳穴分布示意图
(Distribution of auricular points)

1. Sympathetic Nerve
2. External Genitalia
3. Urethra
4. Lower Portion of the Rectum
5. Pharynx
6. External Nose
7. Adrenal
8. Internal Nose
9. Subcortex
10. Esophagus
11. Brainstem

12. Brain Point
13. Ear-Asthma
14. Testis(Ovary)
15. Endocrine
16. Occiput
17. Taiyang
18. Forehead
19. Eye 1
20. Toothache 1
21. Helix 1
22. Shenmen
23. Upper portion of the back
24. Groove for lowering blood pressure
25. Root of the auricular vagus nerve
26. Middle portion of the back
27. Lower portion of the back

 Asthma: Ear-Asthma, Lung, Adrenal.

 Acute sprain or contusion: Auricular point corresponding to the affected area, Subcortex, Ear-Shenmen.

 Dysmenorrhea: Uterus, Endocrine, Liver.

 Acute conjunctivitis: Ear, Liver or Ear Apex.

 Impaired hearing: Internal Ear, Kidney.

 Urticaria: Lung, Liver, Spleen.

常見病症の耳針選穴について（図64）.

頭痛――皮質下、額、枕あるいは太陽。

不眠――神門、心、枕あるいは額、皮質下。

吃逆――膈。

喘息――平喘、肺、腎上腺。

急性捻挫傷――相応部位の耳穴、皮質下、神門。

生理痛――子宮、内分泌、肝。

急性結膜炎――眼、肝あるいは耳尖。

聴力減退――内耳、腎。

蕁麻疹――肺、肝、脾。

下篇 针灸诊疗常用语及词汇

PART C Sentences and Glossary Commonly Used in Acupnucture and Moxibustion during the Consultation Procedure

下篇 針灸の診断治療に常用する言葉および単語

第一节 常用语

I. Common Sentences

第一節 常用する言葉

1. 请坐，您叫什么名字？
   Sit down, please. What is your name?
   どうぞ、おかけください、おなまえはなんとおっしゃいますか。

2. 多大年纪？
   How old are you?
   おいくつですか。

3. 您做什么工作？
   What is your occupation?
   どんなお仕事(しごと)ですか。

4. 您结婚了吗？
   Are you married?
   結婚(けっこん)しておりますか。

5. 您的住址在哪儿？
   What's your address, please?
   御住所(ごじゅうしょ)は。

6. 您哪儿不舒服？请把病情告诉我。
   What's your trouble? Well, tell me about your trouble.
   どこがお悪いですか。病状を云ってください。

7. 我咳嗽的很利害，嗓子疼。
   I have a bad cough and a sore throat.
   せきがひどくて、のどがいたいです。

8. 您过去患过什么病？
   What diseases have you got before?
   いままでに、なにか病気をしたことがありますか。

9. 请告诉我，您过去的病史。
   Please tell me about your past illness.
   今まで、どんな病気をしたか云って下さい。

10. 您这次病多长时间了？
    How long have you been ill?
    この病気にかかってからどのぐらいたちますか。

11. 什么时候痛的更厉害？
    When does your pain become more intense?
    どんな時に痛みが一番ひどいですか。

12. 您现在都有些什么症状？
    What symptoms do you have?

このようにいたくなって、どのぐらいになりますか。

. 胳膊（腿、胸部、腹部）疼吗?
Is there any pain in your arm(leg, chest, abdomen)?
うで（あし、むね、はら）がいたいですか。

20. 是什么样的疼痛，是隐隐约约地疼，还是针扎样疼?
What kind of pain is it ? A dull ache or just a pricking pain?
しくしくいたいのですか、さすようないたみですか。

21. 疼痛和天气（过劳、饮食、情绪）有关吗?
Is there any relation between the pain and the weather (overwork、diet、mood)?
おいたみは、天気（過労、食べ物、気分）と関係がありますか。

22. 您最近的食欲怎样?
How is your appetite recently?
近頃、食欲のほうはいかがですか。

23. 您最近体重减轻吗?
Have you lost any weight recently?
近頃、体重はへっているようですか。

24. 您大便怎样? 多长时间大便一次?
How about your bowel movement? How often do you have your bowels opened?

今は、どんな状態ですか。

13. 您什么地方疼，疼的重吗？
    Where do you feel a pain? Does it hurt yo
    どこがいたいですか。いたみはひどいですか。

14. 请准确地告诉我，哪一个部位觉得疼。
    Show me exactly where you get the pain.
    いたむところを正しく云って下さい。

15. 请用您的手指出哪个地方最疼？
    Point out with your finger where it hurts the most?
    一番痛いところを手でおしえて下さい。

16. 疼痛向别处放散吗？
    Does the pain go anywhere (spread to other parts of the body)?
    痛みは、ほかのところにも出ますか。

17. 这种疼痛是缓慢发生的，还是突然发生的？
    Did pain come on slowly or suddenly?
    いたみは急に出たのですか。それとも、徐徐に痛くなってきたのですか。

18. 您觉得这样疼，有多长时间了？
    How long have you had this pain?

— 297

大便はどうですか。どのぐらいに一回ありますか。

25. 一天排尿几次？
How many times do you urinate a day?
小便は、一日になんかいありますか。

26. 排尿时疼（烧灼感、痒感、刺痛）吗？
Do you have any pain(burning, itching, sharp pain) when you pass water?
小便する時に、いたみ（やくような感じ、かゆい感じ、さすような痛み）がありますか。

27. 您最近感到比以前更容易疲乏吗？
Do you feel more tired than previously?
以前よりつかれやすいですか。

28. 您的月经怎样、量很多吗？
How are your periods? Are they very heavy?
月経はどうですか。量が多いですか。

29. 您有没有查过肝功（血糖、尿糖）？
Have you had your liver function (blood sugar, urine sugar) tested?
肝臓機能（血糖、尿糖）を検査したことがありますか。

30. 您以前用过什么方法治疗（中药、西药、理疗）？

What kind of treatment have you had in the past? (Such as took traditional Chinese medicine, western medicine, physiotherapy.)
以前(いぜん)に、どんな治療をうけましたか。

31. 我给您诊一下脉，请把手放在脉枕上。
Let me feel your pulse. Lay your hand (wrist) on the little pillow.
脈(みゃく)をみてみましょう、手をこの枕(まくら)の上(うえ)にのせて下(くだ)さい。

32. 您的脉有些沉迟（细、弦、滑、数）。
Your pulse is deep and slow (thready, wiry, rolling, rapid).
みゃくは沈遅(ちんち)（細(ほそ)い、弦(げん)、滑(かつ)、数(さく)）ですね。

33. 请把舌头伸出来，再往外伸一点。
Now show me your tongue, push it out a little more.
舌(した)を見(み)せて下(くだ)さい、もうちょっとだしてください。

34. 您的舌苔很厚。
Your tongue is very much coated.
舌苔(ぜったい)が厚(あつ)いですね。

35. 请躺在床上（俯卧、右侧卧、左侧卧）让我给您检查一下。
Please lie down on your back (stomach, right side,

left side)on the bed. Let me examine you.
診察(しんさつ)しますから、ベットのうえによこになって下(くだ)さい
(伏(ふ)せて、右(みぎ)むき、左(ひだり)むき)。

36. 请先把您的双膝屈起来。
Please bend your knees first.
ひざをまげてください。

37. 请躺在床上，放松、两腿分开。
Lie down on this table(bed), please. Relax yourself, spread your legs apart.
ベットによこになって、リラックスして、両(りょう)あしを開(ひら)いてください。

38. 请不要过分注意您的腿，最好随便些。
Don't mind about your legs. You'd better be a little free.
あしにあまり気(き)をつかわずに、気楽(きらく)にしてください。

39. 明天早晨在早饭前到化验室来抽血（化验肝功、空腹血糖）。
Please come to our laboratory tomorrow morning before breakfast to have your blood (liver function, fasting blood sugar)sampled.
明朝(みょうあさ)、朝飯前(あさごはんまえ)に採血(さいけつ)のために来(き)て下(くだ)さい。(肝機能検査(かんきのうけんさ)、空腹時血糖検査(くうふくじけっとうけんさ))

40. 医生，我得的是什么病？

Doctor, what illness have I got?
せんせい。わたしの びょうきはどんな びょうきですか。

41. 你恐怕是得了糖尿病。
I'm afraid you may have diabetes.
とうにょうびょうのようですね。

42. 我该怎么办呢？糖尿病能治好吗？
What should I do? Can diabetes be cured?
どうしたらよいでしょうか。とうにょうびょうはよくなりますか。

43. 我认为最好现在开始给你用饮食疗法和针刺疗法综合治疗。
I think it would probably be wise to start you on a diet at present with acupuncture combination therapy.
いまから しょくじりょうほうと ハリちりょうを いっしょにしたほうが いちばんよいと おもいます。

44. 您的病需要相当长一段时间的治疗。
You need quite a long time for treatment.
あなたの びょうきは、なおるまでに、かなり じかんがかかるかもしれません。

45. 别着急，经过治疗您的病会慢慢好的。
Don't worry. You will gradually get better under the treatment.
あなたの びょうきは、ちりょうしたらだんだんよくなりますから

あせらないでください。

46. 这病不容易好、针灸可能有些效果，但是需要长期治疗。
This kind of disease is difficult to cure, acupuncture may have some effect but prolonged treatment will be needed.
この病気は治りにくいけれども、ハリでよくなるかもしりません。しかし、長い間かかりますよ。

47. 针灸疗法可以治好许多中、西药治不好的病，可以试一试。
Acupuncture and moxibustion therapy can treat many diseases which can't be cured by Chinese medicinal herbs and western medicine. You may have a try.
針灸療法は、漢方薬や西洋薬でなおらない病気を治すことができますから、ためしてみてもいいですよ。

48. 您如愿意，我给您用针刺治疗。
I would like to treat you with acupuncture if you agree.
希望するようでしたら、ハリ療法で治療しましょう。

49. 针灸疗法是中国几千年的经验，效果很好。
Acupuncture and moxibustion therapy have rich experience for thousands of years in China and the effect is quite good.
針灸療法は、中国のなん千年の経験がありますから、

— 303 —

ききめがとてもよいです。

50. 我建议您做一个疗程的针灸治疗。
 I suggest you have a course of acupuncture treatment.
 針灸療法(しんきゅうりょうほう)をひとクールやってみるようにおすすめします。

51. 针灸疗法简便易行、适应症广、无副作用。
 Acupuncture therapy is simple and easy to practise, its indications are wide and there are no side-effects.
 針灸療法(しんきゅうりょうほう)は、簡単(かんたん)でやりやすく、適応症(てきおうしょう)もひろく、副作用(ふくさよう)もありません。

52. 针灸对这种病（腰痛、偏头痛、失眠）最有效。
 Acupuncture is the most effective treatment for this kind of disease (backache, hemicrania, sleeplessness).
 針灸(しんきゅう)は、この病気(びょうき)(腰痛(ようつう)、偏頭痛(へんとうつう)、不眠(ふみん))に対(たい)して、とてもききめがありますよ。

53. 针刺治疗对你的病肯定会有效的。
 I'm sure that acupuncture treatment will help you a great deal.
 あなたの病気(びょうき)は、ハリ治療(ちりょう)で、必(かなら)ずききめがあります。

54. 不要怕，扎针不会叫你疼的。
Don't be afraid.The needles won't hurt you.
針を刺す時いたくありませんから、こわがらないでください。

55. 扎几次针，就能治好您的病。
Several courses of acupuncture treatment will cure you of your illness.
ハリで數回治療したら、あなたの病気はよくなります。

56. 我把针扎到您身上的穴位中去。
I'm going to put needles into certain points on your body.
ハリをツボにさします。

57. 针刺只有轻微的疼痛，或产生一些麻和胀的感觉。
Acupuncture may cause just a little pain,or some feeling of numbness and distension.
ハリをさす時には、かすかないたみ、またはしびれるような感じ、あるいははれぼったような感じがあります。

58. 请解开裤带、脱下外裤（上衣、鞋、袜子）。
Please untie your belt and take off your trousers (jacket,shoes,socks).
バントをゆるめて、ツボンをぬいて下さい（うわぎ、くつ、くつした）。

59. 请把您的右臂放在您的头上。
    Now put your right arm over your head.
    右(みぎ)うでをあたまのうえにのせてください。

60. 不要转头，把头放低一点，靠在椅子上。
    Don't turn your head but lower it a little. Lean on the chair.
    あたまをまわさないようにして、ひくいすのうえにのせてください。

61. 请不要动，也不要紧张。
    Please don't move and take it easy.
    うごかないで、きらくにしてください。

62. 不要紧张，请把肌肉放松。
    Don't be nervous. Relax your muscles, please.
    リラックスして、ちからをぬいてください。

63. 现在看来，你确实有些紧张。
    You do seem rather tense at the moment.
    今(いま)、みると、あなたは、やはり緊張(きんちょう)していますね。

64. 您可以闭上眼睛，不要摒住气。
    You can close your eyes. Don't hold your breath.
    目(め)をとじてもいいですが、息(いき)をころす必要(ひつよう)はありませんよ。

65. 请深呼吸（正常呼吸，轻轻地呼吸）。

Take a deep (normal, soft) breath, please.
深く呼吸（正常呼吸、軽い呼吸）して下さい。

66. 您晕过针吗？
Did you have acupuncture faintness before?
うんしんしたことがありますか。

67. 如果您感到头昏恶心，请告诉我。
If you have faintness and nausea, just let me know.
めまいやおしんがありましたら、すぐおっしゃってください。

68. 针刺这里，您感到疼痛吗？
Do you feel pain when I prick here?
ここをさして、いたいかんじがありますか。

69. 您若感到疼痛，请告诉我。
If you feel a pain tell me, please.
いたいかんじがあったら、おっしゃってください。

70. 我把针扎进去以后，您可能感到发麻。
When I insert the needles into points you may have a feeling of soreness.
ハリをさしたあとに、だるいようなかんじがあるかもしれません。

71. 扎针时您有麻木和发胀的感觉吗？
Do you have the sensation of distension and numb_

ness at needling?

ハリをさすとき、しびれるような感(かん)じ、または張れぼったいようなかんじがありますか。

72. 强烈的胀和麻。
It's intense distension and numbness.
はげしくはれぼったいような感(かん)じとしびれるような感(かん)じがします。

73. 疼痛部位有发凉的感觉吗?
Do you feel cold in the painful place?
いたいところに冷(ひ)えるような感(かん)じがありますか。

74. 您感到下肢发热吗?
Do you feel hot in your legs?
あしにあついようなかんじがありますか。

75. 您不要害怕,只有这样感觉才会有效果。
You needn't worry for only after having such a feeling can it be effective.
このような感(かん)じがあるほうがききめがいいですから、心配(しんぱい)しなくていいですよ。

76. 我捻针时,您有什么感觉。
What do you feel when I rotate the needles?
捻針(ねんしん)するときにどんな感(かん)じがありますか。

77. 捻针时，您会有热（冷）感。
　　You'll have a sense of warmth (coldness) while I'm twisting the needle.
　　捻針する時に熱い（ひえる）感じがありますよ。

78. 我行针时，您会有一种触电样的感觉。
　　You'll have a slight electrical sensation while I'm manipulating the needle.
　　ハリをさす時に、電気にふれたような感じがありますよ。

79. 请躺好，要留针20分钟。
　　Lie down, please. You will have to retain the inserted needle for twenty minutes.
　　にじっ分間留針しますから、横になって、動かないようにしていて下さい。

80. 行针时，请不要动。
　　Don't move when I am manipulating the needle.
　　針刺する時には、動かないでください。

81. 您今天感觉怎么样？
　　How are you feeling today?
　　今日は、感じがどうですか。

82. 我给您取针后，还给您拔几个火罐。
　　I'd like to give you a cupping treatment when the

— 309 —

needles are removed.

ハリをぬきとったあと、火罐(かかん)をいくつかかぶせましょう。

83. 我还可以用电针疗法给您治疗。
I can treat your disease with electro-acupuncture therapy.
また、電針(でんしん)で治療(ちりょう)してあげましょう。

84. 不要害怕，电针只给您一种震颤的感觉。
Don't be afraid. You will only feel a vibrating sensation.
電針(でんしん)は、震(ふる)えるような感(かん)じがあるだけですから、おそれなくてもいいですよ。

85. 这种病可以用埋针的办法治疗。
This kind of disease may be treated with the method of embedded needling.
この病気(びょうき)は、埋針療法(まいしんりょうほう)で治療(ちりょう)することができます。

86. 用耳针治这种病，是一种新方法。
It is a new method for treating the disease with the ear acupuncture.
耳針(じしん)で、この病気(びょうき)を治療(ちりょう)するのは、新(あたら)しい方法(ほうほう)です。

87. 咱们试试艾灸吧，烫时请告诉我。
Let's do some moxibustion. Please let me know if it's too hot.

お灸を試して見ましょう、焼くような感じがあったら、おっしゃってください。

88. 您很合作，非常感谢。
You are most cooperative. Thank you very much.
よく協力してくれました。どうもありがとうございました。

89. 今天就治疗完了，明天上午再来做第2次治疗。
That's all for today. Please come back for the next treatment tomorrow morning.
今日の治療はこれで終ります。あしたの午前に第2回の治療においでください。

90. 我什么时候再来复诊？
When should I come back for the next treatment?
わたしは、この次いつ来たらよいでしょうか。

91. 我们每天针刺1次，共7天，您看行吗？
We will try it every day for seven days, will that be all right?
毎日1回で、7日間つづけて治療する予定です。いいでしょうか。

92. 以后每隔1天，来扎1次针。
Come back for acupuncture every other day.

— 311 —

これから1日おきに1回針治療においでください。

93. 您要隔日来针刺1次,3～4周后就会痊愈的。
You should have acupuncture every other day. You'll be all right within three or four weeks.
1日おきに1回針治療をすれば、3週間か4週間で治ると思います。

94. 针刺治疗一般是每天或隔日1次,10次为1个疗程,每个疗程中间间歇3～5天。
Treatment is given once every day or every other day. Ten treatments make a course. The interval between courses is 3～5 days.
普通は、毎日または隔日1回で、10回をひとクールとします。クールのあいだに3日間ないし5日間休みます。

95. 请您每天到这里来针治1次。
Please come here once a day for acupuncture treatment.
毎日1回針治療においでください。

96. 上次扎针以后,有什么反应?
How did you feel after acupuncture last time?
この前ハリさしたあと、どんな反応がありましたか。

97. 扎针后,您感觉怎样?
How do you feel after acupuncture?

ハリをさしたあと、どんな感[かん]じがありますか。

98. 根据您的情况，我想再做几次治疗，巩固一下疗效为好。
   According to your progress, you'd better have a few more treatments to consolidate the results.
   あなたの場合[ばあい]は、効果[こうか]を高[たか]めるために、あと何回[なんかい]か治療[ちりょう]したほうがいいと思[おも]います。

99. 我想给您停几天针，请1周后再来。
   I am going to stop the acupuncture for a few days. Please come back in a week.
   すこしハリさすのを止[や]めたほうがよいと思[おも]います、一週間[いっしゅうかん]のあとにおいでください。

100. 如果有事，请给我来电话，再见。
   Please phone me if anything happens. See you again.
   何[なに]かご用[よう]がありましたら、電話[でんわ]をください。さようなら。

第二节　词　　汇

II. Glossary

A

abdomen　　　　　n. 腹部

abdominal	a.	腹的，腹部的
abduction	n.	展，外展（作用）
abrupt	a.	突然的，猝然的
accord	n.	一致，调和
of one's own ~		自愿地，主动地
accumulation	n.	积累，积聚
acromioclavicular	a.	肩（峰）锁（骨）的
acromion	n.	肩峰
Adam's apple	n.	喉结
adduct	vt.	使内收
adjacent	a.	邻近的；毗连的；紧接着的
adjust	v.	调整，调节，整顿；校准
adrenal	a. & n.	肾上腺的；肾附近的；肾上腺
advisable	a.	可取的，适当的；贤明的
agape	a. & ad.	（惊奇、害怕得）张大着嘴，目瞪口呆；洞开着，张开着
aggravate	vt.	加重(病情、负担、罪行等),使更恶化
ala	n.	翼，翅
albumin	n.	白朊，白蛋白
alcohol	n. & a.	酒精，乙醇；酒精的；含酒精的
align	v.	（使）成一线，（使）成一行；排队
allergic	a.	过敏性的，变应性的；过敏的
alleviate	vt.	减轻（痛苦等）；缓和
alloy	n.	合金；（金属的）成色，纯度
amenorrhea	n.	经闭
ample	a.	足够的，充分的；宽敞的
anatomical	a.	解剖的；解剖学的
angina	n.	咽峡炎；心绞痛(= ~pectoris)

angle	n.	角，角位；角度，方面
anhidrosis	n.	无汗（症）
ankle	n.	踝；踝节部
anorexia	n.	食欲缺乏，厌食
anterior	a.	前面的；先前的，先于的
anteroinferior	a.	前下的
antihelix	n.	对耳轮
anus	n.	肛门
apathetic	n.	无感觉的，冷淡的，漠然的
apex	n.	顶，顶点
aphasia	n.	失语症
aphonia	n.	失音症
apoplexy	n.	卒中，中风
apparatus	n.	器械，设备，仪器；器官
appetite	n.	食欲，胃口；欲望
applicable	a.	可适用的，能应用的；适当的
arrhythmia	n.	心律不齐
artemisia	n.	艾，艾属植物
artery	n.	动脉
arthralgia	n.	关节痛
arthritis	n.	关节炎
articular	a.	关节的
ascend	v.	登高；上升；攀登
ascending	a.	上行的；向上的
aseptic	a.	防腐的；无菌的；冷漠的
aspect	n.	方位；方面；模样，面貌
asthenia	n.	无力，虚弱，衰弱
asthma	n.	气喘（病）
atrophy	n.	萎缩；虚脱；萎缩症

attach	v.	缚，系；附加
attack	n. & v.	攻击，进攻；（疾病）侵袭，发作
attenuate	v.	（使）变细；（使）变小；（使）减小；（使）减弱
auditory	a.	听觉的；听到的
auricle	n.	耳廓
auricular	a.	耳的；听觉的；耳状的；耳廓的
aware	a.	意识到的，知道的，认识的
axilla	n.	腋下
axillary	a.	腋下的

B

backache	n.	背痛，腰痛
bamboo	n.	竹
bead	n.	有孔之小珠；水泡；滴
belch	vi. & n.	打嗝，嗳气
belly	n.	腹部；腹腔；胃；子宫
	v.	（使）胀满，（使）鼓起
below	prep.	在…的下方，在…以下
	adv.	在下面，在下方
beriberi	n.	脚气（病）
beverage	n.	饮料（如汽水、茶、酒等）
biceps	n.	二头肌
bitter	n. & a.	苦；苦味；痛苦的，有苦味的
bleeding	n. & a.	出血；放血；流血的
blindness	n.	眼睛失明；盲人
night ~		夜盲

blister	n. & vi.	水泡；疱；起水疱；起泡
blunt	a. & n.	不锋利的，钝的；短粗的针
	v.	把…弄钝
blur	v. & n.	弄得模糊不清；模糊一片，污迹
borborygmus	n.	腹鸣
border	n.	边，缘；边沿；边界
breadth	n.	宽度；广度
breech	n.	臀部，屁股
brownish	a.	带褐色的
bruise	n.	青肿，伤痕；擦伤
bulge	n.	凸出部分；膨胀；肿胀
burden	n.	担子；负担，负重
buttock	n.	半边屁股；(复)屁股，臀部

C

calm	a.	沉着的，镇定的；平静的
canthus	n.	眦，眼角
capacity	n.	电容；负载量；能力；容积
cardiac	a. & n.	心脏的；心脏病的；患心脏病的人
cardinal	a.	主要的，基本的
carpal	n. & a.	腕骨；腕的
category	n.	种类，部属；类目
catheter	n.	导(液)管
catheterization	n.	导管插入(术)
caudal	a.	尾的，尾部的
cavum	n.	腔；(空)洞
～ conchae		耳甲腔

cerebrospinal	a.	脑脊髓的
cervical	a.	颈的；子宫颈的
channel	n.	（针灸）经；管
cheek	n.	面颊，脸蛋
chest	n.	胸腔，胸膛
chill	n.	寒冷，寒气；寒战；风寒
choke	v.	闷塞；阻塞；窒息
clarity	n.	清澈；透明；明晰
clavicular	a.	锁骨的
clench	vt.	咬紧（牙关）；握紧（拳头等）
close	vt.	关，闭；封闭；终止
clot	n.	（血等的）凝块；块
cloudiness	n.	模糊不清；多云状态
coarse	a.	粗糙的；粗劣的；粗的；约略的
coating	n.	包被；包衣；外衣；涂层
～ of tongue		舌苔
coccyx	n.	尾骨
coincident	a.	同时发生的，重合的，一致的
collapse	n.	虚脱；萎陷；衰弱；崩溃
collateral	n. & a.	侧突；（针灸）络；侧的，副的
column	n.	柱，支柱；圆柱，柱状物
coma	n.	昏迷；麻木
comatose	a.	昏迷的；麻木的
complexion	n.	肤色（尤指面部肤色），气色；（人的）气质
compress	n.	（止血、消炎用的）敷布，压布
condyle	n.	髁状突，髁
condyloid	a.	髁状的
cone	n.	锥体；锥形物

confusion	n.	混乱；混乱状态；混淆
congenital	a.	（疾病、缺陷等）先天的，天生的
congestion	n.	充血
conjunctivitis	n.	结膜炎
consciousness	n.	意识，知觉；觉悟
constipation	n.	秘结；便秘；呆滞
contracture	n.	挛缩
contraindicate	vt.	禁忌（某种疗法等）
contusion	n.	损伤；挫伤
converge	vi.	会聚，集中
convulsion	n.	惊厥，痉挛
coordination	n.	同等，调整，合作；协调
cornea	n.	角膜
corner	n.	角，犄角
costal	a.	肋骨的
cough	n. & vi.	咳，咳嗽
cramp	n. & v.	（肌肉）痉挛，痛性痉挛；使起痉挛
crease	n.	折缝；折痕；皱纹
transverse ~		横纹
crest	n.	脊突；嵴；顶
criterion	n.	标准，准则，尺度
cross	vt.	使相交，与…相交（叉）；穿过
crus	n.	脚，胫，小腿
crypt	n.	隐窝，腺窝；小囊
cubital	a.	肘的；前膊的；尺骨的
cup	vt.	为……拔火罐，把……置于杯内
cupping	n.	拔火罐
curd	n. & v.	凝乳；凝乳状物；（使）凝结

cushion	n. 垫子；插针的针孔；缓解病痛的药物
cyanosis	n. 发绀，青紫
cymba	n. 艇；舟状物
～conchae	耳甲艇
cystitis	n. 膀胱炎
cysto-	n. 膀胱
～fistulation	膀胱造瘘（术）

D

damp	n. 湿气，潮湿
date	n. 海枣，枣椰子
～stone	枣核
deafness	n. 聋
decubitus	n. 卧位；褥疮
defecate	v. 澄清；提净；通大便；排粪
deficiency	n. 缺乏，不足；缺陷
definite	a. 肯定的；确切的；明确的
deformity	n. 畸形，残废；残缺的东西；畸形的人（或物）
deltoideus	n. 三角肌
demonstrate	vt. 证实；（用实例，实验等）说明；表示
depression	n. 机能降低，抑郁症；凹陷；
nervous ～	神经衰弱
depressive	a. 抑压的；抑郁的；消沉的
dermatology	n. 皮肤学；皮肤病学
despond	vi. 沮丧，泄气，失望
deviation	n. （个体发育的变异中的）离差，

		偏离
diabetes	n.	糖尿病；多尿症
~ insipidus		尿崩症
~ mellitus		糖尿病
diameter	n.	直径，对径；透镜放大的倍数
diaphragm	n.	膈；膈膜
diarrhea	n.	腹泻
differentiation	n.	区别，鉴别
digitus	n.	指(趾)
diminish	v.	减少；变小，缩小
discolo(u)r	v.	（使）变色；（使）褪色，（使）污染
disharmony	n.	不调和，不协调
dispel	vt.	驱散，赶跑；消除，消释
distal	a.	远中的，远侧的；末梢的，末端的
distend	v.	（使）扩张；（使）膨胀，（使）肿胀
distension	n.	扩张；膨胀（作用）
disturbance	n.	（身心等方面的）障碍，失调；干扰
division	n.	分开；分划；分配
dizziness	n.	头晕目眩
dorsolumbar	a.	背腰的
dorsum	n.	背，背部；背状部分
downward	a. & adv.	向下的；向下
drain	vt.	排出（水等液体）；耗尽
dribble	vt.	使点滴流下；使逐渐落下
	n.	点滴；细流；少量

— 321 —

dropping	n.	垂下，落下；点滴
dryness	n.	干，干燥；口渴
dull	a.	呆滞的；迟钝的；阴郁的
dyschesia	n.	大便困难
dysentery	n.	痢疾
dysfunction	n.	机能障碍，机能失调
dysmenorrhea	n.	痛经
dyspnea	n.	呼吸困难
dysuria	n.	排尿困难，尿痛

E

eczema	n.	湿疹
edema	n.	浮肿，水肿
efficacy	n.	功效，效验
elbow	n.	肘
elevate	vt.	抬起；使升高；提高
emaciate	v.	使衰弱，使消瘦，
emergency	n.	紧急情况；突然事件；非常时刻
emission	n.	泄精，泄出
emotional	a.	感情（上）的；（易）激动的；激动人的
empirical	a.	经验主义的；以经验为根据的
endocrine	n.	内分泌（腺）；激素
endogenous	a.	内源的，内生的；内源代谢的
enhance	vt.	提高，增加；增强，增进
entangle	vt.	缠住；使纠缠；牵连，使卷入

enuresis	n.	遗尿
epicondyle	n.	上髁
epidemic	a. & n.	流行性的，传染的；流行病，时疫
epigastric	a.	腹上部的，腹部的
epigastrium	n.	腹上部
epilepsy	n.	癫痫，羊痫疯
epistaxis	n.	鼻衄
erect	a.	直立的，竖直的；勃起的
	v.	使竖立；(使)勃起
erode	v.	腐蚀；侵蚀；腐蚀成，受腐蚀
essence	n.	本质，质体；实体；精华，精髓
etiology	n.	病原学，病因学
exacerbation	n.	加剧，加重，恶化
excessive	a.	过多的，过分的；极度的
exertion	n.	尽力，努力；行使
exhaustion	n.	耗尽；枯竭；筋疲力尽
exogenous	a.	外因的；外源的
exophthalmos	n.	突眼症；眼球突出症
expectoration	n.	痰，咳出物；咳出，吐痰
exposure	n.	曝露；暴露；方位
extensor	n.	伸肌
extraordinary	a.	非常的，特别的，离奇的；
extremity	n.	末端；尽头；(身体的)一肢；(人的)手，足
eyebrow	n.	眉；眉毛
eyelid	n.	眼睑

F

f(a)ecal	a.	粪便的;糟粕的;渣滓的
facial	a.	面部的,面部用的
facilitate	vt.	使容易,使便利;推进,促进
faint	n. & vi.	昏厥,晕倒
	a.	虚弱的;衰弱的
famish	v.	(使)挨饿;饥饿
febrile	a.	热病的
feces	n.	粪;排泄物;渣滓
feeble	a.	虚弱的,无力的,微弱的
femur	n.	股骨;大腿
ferment	v.	(使)发酵;(使)激动
	n.	酶,发酵,激动
fetid	a.	恶臭的,腥臭的
fetus	n.	胎,胎儿
fever	n.	发热,发烧;热度;热病
	v.	(使)发烧,(使)患热病
feverish	a.	发烧的,有热病症状的,容易引起热病的
fibrous	a.	含纤维的;纤维状的;纤维构成的
fibula	n.	腓骨
filiform	a.	丝状的;线状的;纤维状的
~ needle		毫针
fine	a.	优秀的;精制的;纤细的,锋利的
fist	n.	拳(头);抓住
fistula	n.	瘘;瘘管
fistulation	n.	成瘘;造瘘术

flabby	a.	(肌肉等)不结实的,松弛的;软弱的
flaccid	a.	(肌肉等)松弛的,不结实的;软弱的
flex	v. & n.	屈曲;折曲
flexible	a.	柔韧的,易弯曲的;可变通的,灵活的
flexion	n.	弯曲;弯曲部分
flexor	n.	屈肌
flush	v.	使(脸等)涨红;(使)脸上发红
	n.	红光;红晕;兴奋;激动
fold	v. & n.	折迭;对折;折,褶
fontanel(le)	n.	囟门
forceps	n.	(单复数同)镊子,钳子
forearm	n.	前臂
forehead	n.	额;前部
forgetfulness	n.	健忘;不注意,疏忽
formula	n.	公式;方案;处方
fossa	n.	窝,凹
nasal ～		鼻凹
foul	a.	(味道)难闻的,恶臭的;腐烂发臭的
frenulum	n.	系带
frequency	n.	屡次,频繁;次数
frontal	a. & n.	前面的,正面的;前额的;额骨
frown	v. & n.	皱眉,蹙额;(用皱眉,蹙额)表示不满

fungus	n.	真菌；海绵肿
fur	n. & vi.	舌苔；水锈；生苔
furuncle	n.	疖（疔疮）

G

gall	n.	胆汁；胆；胆囊；苦味
~ stone		胆石
gastralgia	n.	胃痛
gastric	a.	胃的
gastrocnemius	n.	腓肠肌
gauze	n.	（棉、丝等织成的）薄沙；沙布（金属、塑料等的）网纱
genitalia	n.	生殖器
gentian	n.	龙胆；龙胆属植物
~ violet		龙胆紫
giddiness	n.	眩晕；眼花缭乱
ginger	n.	姜，生姜
gingival	a.	齿龈的，龈的；齿槽的
girdle	n.	带；腰带，围绕物；环形物
glabella	n.	眉间
glossoplegia	n.	舌麻痹
goiter	n.	甲状腺肿；气瘿
govern	v.	统治，管理；指导；支配；决定；影响
grain	n.	谷物，谷类；谷粒；细粒
gravel	n.	砂砾，砾石；尿砂
groove	n.	（器官、骨的）沟；槽
ground	a.	磨过的，磨碎的；(grind 的过去式和过去分词)

gum	n.	齿龈；牙床
gurgle	vi. & n.	（人）发咯咯声；作咕嘟声
gyn(a)ecology	n.	妇科学

H

hack	vi.	断续地干咳　n. 干咳
hairline	n.	头型轮廓，发型轮廓；发际
halitosis	n.	口臭
hallux	n.	蹈趾，蹈
hazard	n.	机会；偶然的事；危险
heel	n.	脚后跟，踵
helix	n.	耳轮
hemafecia	n.	便血
hematemesis	n.	呕血
hematoma	n.	血肿
hematuria	n.	血尿
hemicrania	n.	偏头痛
hemiplegia	n.	偏瘫，半身不遂
hemoptysis	n.	咯血；咳血
hemorrhage	n. & vi.	出血
hemorrhoid	n.	痔
hemostasis	n.	止血（法）
hernia	n.	疝（气），突出
herpes	n.	疱疹
hiatus	n.	裂缝；空隙；中断
hiccup	n. & vi.	打嗝儿，打呃声；打呃
hidrosis	n.	排汗（作用）；多汗；出汗
hip	n.	臀部；髋，髋部
hoarseness	n.	（声音）嘶哑；嗓门嘶哑；暴瘖

horizantal	a.	水平的；地平的，地平线的；卧式的
hormone	n.	激素，荷尔蒙，内分泌
humerus	n.	肱骨
hyoid	n. & a.	舌骨；舌骨的；舌形的
hyperactivity	n.	活动过强；机能亢进
hypersomnia	n.	睡眠过度
hyperthyroidism	n.	甲状腺机能亢进
hypochondriac	a.	季肋部的
hypochondrium	n.	季肋部
hysteria	n.	癔病；歇斯底里

I

ignite	v.	点燃，点火于；使燃烧；使灼热
iliac	a.	髂的，肠骨的
imbalance	n.	不平衡，不均衡
impairment	n.	削弱，损害，损伤
impotence	n.	虚弱，无力；阳痿
inch	n.	英寸
incontinence	n.	失禁，无节制
index	n.	食指；索引
indication	n.	适应症；指征，表示；迹象
indigestion	n.	消化不良，胃弱
infantile	a.	婴儿（期）的，幼儿（期）的，早期的，初期的
infarction	n.	梗塞，梗死；梗塞形成
inferior	a.	（位置）下方的，下部的；在下的；下后的

infrascapular	a.	肩胛下的
infusion	n.	注入，灌输；输注
inherit	vt.	继承；经遗传而得（性格、特征等）
initial	a.	最初的，开始的
inner	n. & a.	内部，里面；内部的；里面的
insert	v.	插进，嵌入；(肌肉)附着
insidious	a.	(疾病) 不知不觉之间加剧的，暗中为害的
insipid	a.	无味的；枯燥乏味的；无生气的
insomnia	n.	失眠，失眠症
insufficiency	n.	不充分，不足；不适当，不胜任；机能不全
intensify	v.	加强；加剧；强化
intercostal	a.	脉间的，脊间的
intermittent	a.	间歇性的，断断续续的，周期性的
interphalangeal	a.	指（趾）节间的
interrogation	n.	讯问，质问
intertragicus	n.	耳屏间肌
intestine	n. & a.	肠；内部的
intolerance	n.	不容忍；不容异说；偏执；不耐
intoxicate	vt.	使喝醉；使陶醉；使中毒
invasion	n.	入侵；侵害；发病，发作
involuntary	a.	非自愿的；非故意的；无意识的；不自觉的
iodine	n.	碘；碘酊
irascibility	n.	性情暴躁；易怒

irregular	a.	不规则的，无规律的
irritability	n.	易怒，烦躁；过敏；应激性
itch	n. & vi.	痒，疥疮；发痒；渴望
itching	a.	痒的；渴望的

J

jar	n.	罐子；广口瓶
jaundice	n.	黄疸
jaw	n.	颌，颚
joint	n.	关节
junction	n.	连结；接合点

K

kidney	n.	肾，腰子；脾气，性格
knead	vt.	揉，捏，按摩（肌肉等）
knee	n.	膝；膝盖；膝关节

L

labo(u)r	n.	分娩，阵痛
lacrimation	n.	流泪
lactation	n.	乳汁的分泌；哺乳
landmark	n.	显而易见的目标；界标
lassitude	n.	疲乏，无力；厌倦，无精打采
lateral	a.	侧面的；旁边的；横（向）的
laxity	n.	松弛，无紧张
lethargy	n.	嗜眠症；昏睡；冷淡；懒散
leukorrhagia	n.	白带过多
leukorrhea	n.	白带

level	n. & a.	水平面；水平；标准；水平的
ligament	n.	韧带
listlessness	n.	倦怠；无精打采
lobule	n.	小叶
locality	n.	位置；地点；发生地，所在地
location	n.	位置；定位
longitudinal	a.	经度的；纵的
longus	a. & n.	长的，长肌
loose	a. & vt.	松的；松散的；把…放开
lower	a.	较低的，下部的
lumbago	n.	腰部风湿痛
lumbar	a. & n.	腰的，腰部的；腰神经，腰椎
lumbosacral	a.	腰骶的
lustre	n.	光泽；光辉；光彩
lustrous	a.	（带有）光泽的，有光彩的，
lymphangitis	n.	淋巴管炎

M

majority	n.	大多数；半数以上
malar	a. & n.	颧骨的，颊的；颧骨
malaria	n.	疟疾
malleolus	n.	踝
mammilla	n.	乳头
mammillary	a.	乳头的；乳头状的
mandible	n.	下颌骨
mandibular	a.	下颌（骨）的
mania	n.	躁狂症；疯狂；癖好

manic	a. & n.	躁狂的；躁狂者
manifestation	n.	表明；现象；表现形式
manipulate	vt.	熟练地使用，操作；处理；处置
manipulation	n.	操作，操纵；处理；手法，操作法
margin	n.	边缘；界限；差数
massage	n. & vt.	按摩；推拿
masseter	n.	咬肌
mastitis	n.	乳腺炎，乳房炎
mastoid	a. & n.	乳头状的；颞骨状突起的；乳突
medial	a.	中间的，居中的；平均的
melancholy	n. & a.	忧郁；忧郁症；意气消沉的；使人抑郁的
memory	n.	记忆，记忆力
meningitis	n.	脑（脊）膜炎
menorrhagia	n.	月经过多
menorrhalgia	n.	痛经
menorrhea	n.	月经过多；行经；月经
menstrual	a.	每月一次的，月经的
menstruation	n.	月经；行经；行经期
mental	a.	精神的；内心的；脑力的；精神病的
mentolabial	a.	颏唇的
metacarpal	a. & n.	掌的；掌骨
metacarpophalangeal	a.	掌骨与指骨的
metatarsal	a. & n.	跖的；跖骨
micturition	n.	排尿
midline	n.	中线
midpoint	n.	中点；中心点
midway	n. & a.	中途，半路；中途的

millet	n.	黍，稷，小米
minimize	vt.	使减到最小，把…估计得最低
minute	a.	微小的，微细的；精密的；仔细的
moderate	a.	中等的，适度的；有节制的
moist	a.	湿性的，有分泌物的；潮湿的；含泪的
monoxide	n.	一氧化物
morphological	a.	形态（学）的
motor	a.	运动的；原动的
mouth	n.	口，口腔，嘴
moxa	n.	艾；艾绒
~ -wool		艾绒
moxibustion	n.	艾灸，艾灼；（艾）灸术
mucoid	a.	粘液样的
mucus	n.	由粘膜分泌的粘液
mugwort	n.	艾蒿
mulberry	n.	桑树；桑属植物；桑子
multipara	n.	经产妇，非初产妇
mumps	n.	流行性腮腺炎
muscle	n.	肌肉；肌
muscular	a.	肌的；肌肉的；强健的；强有力的
muteness	n.	哑；缄默；（一时）说不出话
myasthenia	n.	肌无力，肌衰弱
~ gravis		重症肌无力
myatrophy	n.	肌萎缩
myelitis	n.	脊髓炎；骨髓炎
myocardial	a.	心肌的

N

nail	n.	（手、脚的）指甲；爪
nape	n.	项，项背，后颈
nasal	a. & n.	鼻的；鼻音的；鼻骨
nasolabial	a.	鼻唇的
nausea	n.	恶心；晕船
neck	n.	颈，脖子
needle	n. & vt.	针；用针刺
nervous	a.	神经的；神经方面的；紧张不安的
neuralgia	n.	神经痛
neurology	n.	神经病学
neurosis	n.	神经（机能）病，精神神经病
nipple	n.	乳头
nocturnal	a.	夜的；夜间发生的；夜间活动的
notch	n.	凹口，槽口
numbness	n.	麻木；失去感觉

O

obliquely	ad.	斜地，倾斜地；偏斜地
obstetric(al)	a.	产科（学的）助产的
obstruction	n.	阻塞，堵塞；阻碍
occipital	a.	枕骨的
occiput	n.	枕（骨）部
odour	n.	气味；香气；臭气；味道
ophthalmalgia	n.	眼痛
ophthalmology	n.	眼科学
ophthalmopathy	n.	眼病

ophthalmoplegia	n.	眼肌麻痹
opisthotonos	n.	角弓反张
orbit	n.	眼窝，眼眶
orbital	a.	眼窝的，眶的；轨道的
original	a.	原来的，固有的；最初的，最早的
otolaryngology	n.	耳鼻喉科学
otorrhea	n.	耳液溢
overcast	a.	多云的，阴暗的；郁闷的

P

pain	vi. & n.	作痛，觉得痛；疼痛
palate	n.	腭
pallor	n.	（脸色等的）苍白，灰白
palm	n.	手掌，手心
palmar	a.	掌中的；手掌的
palmaris	n.	掌肌
palpitation	n.	心悸；跳动
panic	n. & a.	恐慌，惊慌，恐慌的
papular	a.	丘疹的
papule	n.	丘疹
paralysis	n.	麻痹；瘫痪
paraphasia	n.	语言无序，语言错乱
paraphobia	n.	轻（度）恐怖
paraphronia	n.	性情变易
parietal	a.	体壁的；腔壁的；顶骨的
paroxysmal	a.	发作性的，阵发的；爆发性的
patella	n.	髌，膝盖（骨）；膝节
pathogenic	a.	病原的，致病的；发病的
pathological	a.	病理学的；由疾病引起的；病态的

pediatrics	n.	儿科学，小儿科
pedis	n.	足
peevish	a.	易怒的，暴躁的；倔强的；带怒气的
pelvis	n.	骨盆
penetration	n.	穿入，穿透；穿透能力
penis	n.	阴茎
periauricular	a.	耳廓周的；心房周的
perineum	n.	会阴
period	n.	时期；时代；期，周期；月经期
peronaeus	n.	腓骨肌
perpendicularly	ad.	垂直地
perspiration	n.	汗；出汗
petechia	n.	瘀点，瘀斑
philtrum	n.	人中（鼻唇间纵沟）
phlegm	n.	痰；粘液，迟钝，冷淡
phonate	vi.	发音；发出语音
photophobia	n.	畏光；羞明
physiotherapy	n.	物理疗法，理疗
pinch	vt.	捏；轧痛，使不舒服，使萎缩
pink	n. & a.	桃红色，粉红色；粉红色的
pisiform	n. & a.	豌豆骨；豌豆骨的
plantar	a.	蹠的，脚底的
polydipsia	n.	烦渴
polyorexia	n.	过饥，善饥
polyphagia	n.	贪食（症）；杂食；混食
polypus	n.	息肉
polyuria	n.	多尿（症）
Popliteal	a.	腘的

posterior	a.	后面的，其次的
postpartum	a.	产后的
potential	n.	（电）位，势；潜势；可能（性）
precaution	n. & vt.	预防；警惕；预防方法；使提防
precede	vt.	先于…，位于…之前；比…优先；在…前加上；
pregnancy	n.	怀孕，怀胎；怀孕期
premenstrual	a.	月经前的
prescription	n.	药方，处方；处方的药
presentation	n.	先露，产式
prevalent	a.	流行的；盛行的，普遍的
prick	n. & vt.	刺痛；刺，穿
probe	n. & vt.	探针；探查，探索；
process	n.	进程；变化的过程；隆起，突
prodrome	n.	前驱症状；序论
profuse	a.	过多的；极其丰富的，充沛的
prolapse	n.	脱出症，脱垂，下垂
prolong	vt.	延长；拉长；拖延
prominence	n.	显著；凸出；突起
promote	v.	促进；发扬；引起
prone	a.	俯伏的，面向下的；倾斜的
pronounced	a.	显著的，明确的；发出音的
prophylaxis	n.	预防；预防法
proportional	a.	成比例的；相称的，均衡的
prospermia	n.	早泄，射精过早
protract	vt.	延长，拖延
protrude	v.	（使）伸出，（使）突出；耸出
protuberance	n.	隆起；突出物；隆起部；疙瘩

proximal	a.	最接近的；近侧的，近身体中心（或关节）的
pruritus	n.	瘙痒
psychiatry	n.	精神病学
psychotic	a.	精神病的；患精神病的
	n.	精神病患者
ptosis	n.	下垂；
pubis	n.	耻骨
puncture	v. & n.	（用针）刺；刺，穿刺；扎
purple	n. & a.	紫色，紫红色；紫的，紫红的
purulent	a.	化脓的；脓性的；含脓的
pustula	n.	脓疱
pustular	a.	小脓疱的；小脓疱状的；生小脓疱的
pustule	n.	小脓疱；小疱
pyogenic	a.	生脓的

Q

qi(vital energy)	n.	气
quadriceps	n.	四头肌

R

radial	a.	桡骨的；辐射状的
radiate	v.	散发，传播；辐射状发出
radius	n.	桡骨；半径
rattle	n.	啰音；喉部发出的哮吼声
realm	n.	领域，范围；类；门
recipe	n.	处方；配方；方法
rectum	n.	直肠

recumbent	a.	躺着的；斜靠的；横卧的，斜倚的
recurrent	a.	再发的；经常发生的；周期性发生的
redness	n.	红，赤色
reflex	vt. & n.	使经历反射过程；把…折回；反射
region	n.	部，部位，范围；地区
regurgitation	n.	回流；反胃，回吐
reinforce	vt.	加强；支援；增援；增加…的数量（或厚度）
relaxed	a.	松懈的；放松的；随意的，不拘束的
remote	a.	相隔很远的，遥远的；偏僻的
removal	n.	移动；除掉，切除；排除
repetition	n.	重复；反复
respective	a.	各自的，各个的
retention	n.	停滞，固位；保持；保留
rheumatic	n. & a.	风湿病患者；（患）风湿病的
rheumatism	n.	风湿病
rheumatoid	a.	风湿病的；类风湿病的
rhinitis	n.	鼻炎
rhinorrhea	n.	鼻（液）溢
rib	n.	肋，肋骨；
rigidity	n.	刚硬，坚硬；僵化；严格
rim	n.	（圆形器皿的）边，缘
rolling	a.	滚（动）的；周而复始的；摇摆的
rotate	v.	（使）旋转；（使）转动；（使）循环

rubella	n.	风疹
rubeola	n.	麻疹；风疹

S

sacral	a.	骶的；荐骨的
sacrum	n.	骶骨；荐骨
saline	n.	盐水
salivation	n.	多涎，过量的唾液分泌
sallow	a.	（人、肤色）灰黄色的，菜色的
scalp	n.	（人的）头皮
scanty	a.	不充足的；贫乏的；狭小的；稀疏的
scapha	n.	耳舟
scapula	n.	肩胛（骨）；肩板
schizophrenia	n.	精神分裂症
sciatic	a.	坐骨的；臀部的，坐骨神经痛的
sciatica	n.	坐骨神经痛
sclera	n.	（眼球的）巩膜
scrofula	n.	瘰疬，淋巴结核
seizure	n.	（疾病的）发作
seminal	a.	精液的；生殖的
semitendinosus	n.	半腱肌
sensation	n.	感觉，知觉，激动
sensitive	a.	敏感的；容易感受的，神经过敏的
severe	a.	严重的；剧烈的；严厉的
shortness	n.	短；矮；缺乏，简短
shoulder	n.	肩，肩膀；肩膀关节
sign	n.	征兆；迹象；（病）症

simplicity	n.	简单；简易；简明；单纯
slightly	ad.	轻微地；少量地；微小地
slippery	a.	滑的；使人滑跤的；易滑脱的；含糊的
smash	vt.	打碎，打破；粉碎
sniffle	vi.	（一再）抽鼻子；发声地吸气；抽着鼻子说话
soak	v.	浸，泡，(使)浸透
sole	n.	脚底，鞋底；基底
somnolence	n.	嗜眠（症）；思睡，困倦
soothe	vt.	安慰；使平静；使（痛苦，疼痛等）减轻
space	n.	空间；间隔，距离
spasm	n.	痉挛，抽搐；(动作、感情等的)一阵发作
spina	n.	脊柱；脊髓；
～ bifida		脊椎裂
spine	n.	脊柱；脊骨；类似脊骨的东西
spinous	a.	棘状的；刺的；棘突的
spontaneous	a.	自发的；本能的；自动的
spot	n.	点；斑点，疵点，污点
sprain	vt. & n.	扭伤，扭
sputum	n.	唾沫，痰
stab	v. & n.	刺，刺入；尝试
stagnate	v.	（使）停滞，（使）不流动，（使）迟钝
stainless	a.	不锈的；没有污点的；纯洁的
stasis	n.	壅滞，郁积，停滞
stem	n.	茎；(树)干；(叶)梗

stenocardia	n.	心绞痛
sterile	a.	无菌的；消过毒的
sterility	n.	不育，不孕；无菌（状态）；无效
sterilize	vt.	把…消毒，使无菌；使绝育
sternocleidomastoideus	n.	胸锁乳突肌
sternocostal	a.	胸肋的；胸骨和肋骨的
sternum	n.	胸骨
sticky	a.	粘性的；胶粘的；湿热的；痛苦的
stiffness	n.	硬；僵直；僵硬；不灵活
stifle	v.	使窒息；使闷住；闷死；受抑制
stifling	a.	令人窒息的，气闷的；沉闷的
stir	v.	动；移动；摇动；激起；活动
stomatitis	n.	口炎
stomatology	n.	口腔学
stool	n.	大便，粪便
strain	n.	拉紧；过劳；极度紧张；扭伤
stranguria	n.	疼痛性尿淋沥；淋证
stress	n.	压力，重压；紧迫；紧张；强调
stretch	v.	伸展；延伸；使（精神、肌肉等）过度紧张
strike	vt.	打；击；撞击；（疾病）侵袭
stroke	n.	打击；（病）突然发作；中风；麻痹
styloid ～ process	a.	柱状的 茎突
subcortex	n.	下皮质；皮质下部

subglossal	a.	舌下的
subjective	a.	主观的；自觉的
submandibular	a.	下颌下的
suck	v.	吸，吮；吸收，吸取
suction	n.	吸，吸入（排去空气后所产生的）吸力
suffocate	v.	（使）窒息；把…闷死
sunstroke	n.	中暑，日射病
superficial	a.	表面的，表面性的；快而粗略的
superior	a.	（指位置方面）在上的，较高的
supraorbital	a.	眶上的
suprasternal	a.	胸骨上的
surgery	n.	外科手术；外科；外科学
suspicious	a.	可疑的；多疑的；猜疑的
swab	vt.	（用药签）敷药于；（用拭子等）拭抹
swallow	v. & n.	吞下，咽下；吞；咽喉
sweat	n.	汗；出汗；焦躁
swelling	n. & a.	肿胀，肿大，肿大的；突起的
swift	a.	快的；突然发生的；反应快的
swiftly	ad.	迅速地；敏捷地
symmetrically	ad.	对称地；匀称地
sympathetic	a.	交感（神经系）的；同情的
symphysis	n.	（骨的）联合（线）
symptom	n.	症状，征兆，征候
syncope	n.	昏厥
syndrome	n.	综合征，症候群
syringe	n.	注射器；洗涤器
	vt.	（用注射器等）注射

T

taste	n.	味觉；味道，滋味
tastelessness	n.	无味
temporal	a.	太阳穴的，颞颥的
tender	a.	敏感的；一触即痛的
tendon	n.	腱
tenesmus	n.	里急后重；下坠；后坠
tense	a.	拉紧的，绷紧的，紧张的
tetanic	a.	破伤风性的，强直性痉挛的
therapeutic	a.	治疗（学）的，疗法的
thigh	n.	股，大腿
thoracic	a.	胸的，胸廓的
thready	a.	纤细的，纤细无力的；线状的
three-edged needle	n.	三棱针
throbbing	a.	跳动的，悸动的；抽动的（有规律地）颤动的
thrust	v.	插；塞；刺；戳；延伸
thumb	n.	（大）拇指
tibia	n.	胫骨
tilt	vt.	使倾斜；使翘起
tingle	v.	（使）感刺痛，（耳等）鸣响；震颤
tinnitus	n.	耳鸣
tip	n.	梢，末梢；尖，尖端
tipsy	a.	喝醉的；醉醺醺的
toe	n.	脚趾；足尖
tongue	n.	舌，舌头
touch	vt.	触摸；接触，碰到；轻按

toothache	n.	牙痛
tragus	n.	耳屏，耳珠
trance	n.	恍惚，出神；发呆；迷睡
transient	a.	短暂的，易逝的；无常的
transverse	n. & a.	横骨，横肌；横向的，横切的
trapezius	n.	斜方肌
trauma	n.	损伤，外伤
tremor	n.	震颤；发抖；震动，微动
trigeminal	a.	三叉神经的
trismus	n.	牙关紧闭
trochanter	n.	转子
turbid	a.	混浊的，污浊的；混乱的
twirl	vt.	使快速转动，使快速旋转；捻弄
twitch	v.	（肌肉等）颤动，抽搐；抽痛，阵痛

U

ulcerous	a.	患溃疡的，溃疡（性）的
ulna	n.	尺骨
ulnar	a.	尺骨的，尺侧的
umbilicus	n.	脐；中心
upward	a. & ad.	向上的；上升的；向上
urethra	n.	尿道
urethralgia	n.	尿道痛
urinary	a.	尿的；泌尿的，泌尿器的
urine	n.	尿
urticaria	n.	风疹，荨麻疹
uterine	a.	子宫的
uterus	n.	子宫

V

vacuum	v.	真空;真空般状态
vegetative	a.	生长性的;植物性的;植物的
vein	n.	静脉,(俗)血管
vertebra	n.	椎骨,脊椎
vertex	n.	顶点,顶,头顶
vertical	a.	垂直的;竖式的;头顶的
vertigo	n.	眩晕;头晕
vesicle	n.	囊;泡;水疱
vibrate	v.	(使)颤动;(使)震动
vice	prep.	代替,接替
～ versa		反过来,(也是这样)
vicinity	n.	附近,近处
vigorously	ad.	强有力地;壮健地,精力充沛地
viscera	n.	内脏,脏腑;内容
vision	n.	视,视力,视觉
vital	a.	生命的,生机的,有生命力的;致命的;极其重要的
voluntary	a.	由主观意志决定的;随意的,自发的
vomiting	n.	呕吐
vulgaris	a.	寻常的;普通的
vulva	n.	外阴,女阴,阴门

W

watery	a.	水的,湿的;象水的,稀薄的
weakness	n.	虚弱;软弱;癖好
web	n.	蛛网状组织;蹼

wheal	n.	风块，荨麻疹团；疱，水疱
wheat	n.	小麦
whirl	v.	（使）回旋；（使）旋转；发晕
whitish	a.	带白色的；有些苍白的
width	n.	宽阔；广博，宽度，阔度
wiry pulse	n.	弦脉
withdrawal	n.	收回，撤回；停止服药
worsen	v.	（使）变得更坏，（使）恶化，损害
wrap	v.	环绕；覆盖；遮蔽
wrist	n.	腕；腕关节

X

xu(deficiency or insufficiency)	n.	虚

Y

yellowish	a.	带黄色的，淡黄色的

Z

zoster	n.	带状疱疹
zygomatic	a.	颧骨的；颧的

第二節　単　語※

あ

あおそこひ	青底翳（青光眼）
あかあざ	赤痣（血管痣）
あかい	赤い（红）
あかはな	赤鼻（酒糟鼻）
あかめ	赤目（結膜炎）
アキレスけん	（跟腱）
あくび	欠伸（呵欠）
あしのけついんかんけい	足厥陰肝経
あしのしょういんじんけい	足少陰腎経
あしのしょうようたんけい	足少陽胆経
あしのたいいんひけい	足太陰脾経
あしのたいようぼうこうけい	足太陽膀胱経
あしのようめいいけい	足陽明胃経
あぜけつ	阿是穴
あつくねばりけがある	厚く粘り気がある（厚膩）

い

いかんつう	胃脘痛
いきぎれ	息切れ（呼吸困难）
いきふわ	胃気不和
いきょじゅかん	胃虚受寒
いしきもうろう	意識朦朧
いしょう	萎症（痿证）

いせい	遺精
いたみ	痛み（痛感）
いちふほう	一夫法
いちゅう	委中
いつう	胃痛
いにょう	遺尿
いびき	鼾
いぼ	疣
いんい	陰萎（阳痿）
いんこうしゅつう	咽喉腫痛
いんしょくていたい	飲食停滞
いんどう	印堂
いんぱく	隠白
いんぶつう	陰部痛
いんりょうせん	陰陵泉

う

うすい	薄い（薄）
うすしろい	薄白い（薄白）
うで	腕（臂）
うなじ	項
うみ	膿
うわごと	譫語
うんしん	暈針

え

えいふう	翳風
えけつ	会穴
えくぼ	笑窪（酒窩）

えんげしょうがい	嚥下障碍（咽下困难）

お

おいる	老いる（衰老）
おうととまらず	嘔吐止まらず（呕吐不止）
おうだん	黄疸
おうもん	横紋
おかん	悪寒
おけつ	瘀血
おくび	噯気
おたふくかぜ	お多福風（流行性腮腺炎）
おふう	悪風
おりもの	下り物（白帯）

か

かいけい	解谿
がいかん	外関
がいかん	艾巻
がいがんかくつう	外眼角痛（外眦痛）
がいせいしょくきとうつう	外生殖器疼痛
がいそう	咳嗽
がいちゅう	艾柱
がいちゅうきゅう	艾柱灸
がいしょう	外傷
がいじゅう	艾絨
がいじょう	艾条
かいぼうひょうきほう	解剖標記法
かくえんきゅう	隔塩灸
かくきょうきゅう	隔姜灸

かくにんきゅう	隔蒜灸
かくへいきゅう	隔餅灸
かくゆ	膈俞
かしのきんにくいしゅく	下肢の筋肉萎縮(下肢萎缩)
かがとのいたみ	踵の痛み（足跟痛）
かしまひ	下肢麻痺
かぜ	風邪（感冒）
かた	肩
かた、うでそうごうぐん	肩手症候群（肩手综合征）
かだきょうせき	華佗夾脊
かたこり	肩凝り（凝肩）
かっけつ	喀血
かっさく	滑数
かのうきゅう	化膿灸
かるいもの	軽いもの（轻者）
かれごえ	枯聲（嘶哑）
かんがいむたん	乾咳無痰
かんきはんい	肝気犯胃
かんきゅう	顴弓
がんけんけいれん	眼瞼痙攣（眼睑瞤动）
かんげん	関元
かんし	間使
かんしつ	寒湿
かんしつげり	寒湿下利
かんじゃないせき	寒邪内積
かんちょう	環跳
かんぼう	感冒
かんゆ	肝俞
かんようじょうこう	肝陽上亢

がんめんふしゅ	顔面浮腫
がんめんしんけいまひ	顔面神経麻痺

き

きえ	気会
きえい	気癭
きかい	気海
きけい	奇経
きけいはちみゃく	奇経八脈
きけつ	気穴
きけつ	気血
きけつふそく	気血不足
きけつりょうきょ	気血両虚
きし	気至
きちがい	気違い（精神病）
きもん	期門
きはく	稀薄
きゅうきょうふう	急驚風
きゅうほう	灸法
きゅうり	久痢
きょ	虚
きょうき（けいき）	驚悸
きょうけつ	驚厥
きょうふ	僵撲
きょうしょう	狂症
きょうつう	脇痛
きょかん	虚寒
きょくち	曲池
ぎょさい	魚際

きょさく	虚数
きょじゃく	虚弱
きょひ	虚秘
きりきりいたい	きりきり痛い（微痛）
きんしん　ぎょくえき	金津　玉液

く

くだる	下る（腹瀉）
くちがにがい	口が苦い（口苦）
くちのくさみ	口の臭み（口臭）
くろめ	黒目（瞳孔）

け

けいき	経気
けいき（きょうき）	驚悸
けいけつ	榮穴
けいけつ	経穴
げいこう	迎香
けいこうきょうつう	頸項強痛
けいこうぶつう	頸項部痛
けいこく	谿谷
けいつい	経隧
けいみゃく	経脈
けいらく	経絡
げかん	下関
けつ	穴
けつい	穴位
けつえ	血会
けっかい	血海

げっけいかた	月経過多
げっけいへいし	月経閉止
げっけいふじゅん	月経不順（月经不调）
けつどう	穴道
けつまくえん	結膜炎
げねつ	解熱
げり	下痢
げんうん	眩暈
けんおん	検温
けんぐう	肩髃
げんけつ	原穴
けんこうつう	肩甲痛
げんごむりょく	言語無力
けんてい	肩貞
けんしょう	懸鐘
けんはくけいれん	肩膊痙攣
けんぼう	健忘
けんわんつう	肩腕痛

こ

こうかくのゆがみ	口角の歪み（囗角歪斜）
こうかつ	口渇
こうかん	行間
こうがんのゆがみ	口眼の歪み（口眼歪斜）
こうき	候気
こうき	後期
こうぎ	講義（讲授）
こうけい	後谿
ごうけつ	合穴

こうこうかいよう	口腔潰瘍
ごうこく	合谷
こうしゅう	口臭
こうじ	黄膩
ごうしん	毫針
こうぶきょうちょく	項部強直
こつえ	骨会
こつどぶんすんほう	骨度分寸法
こつじょうちょうねつ	骨蒸潮熱
こむらがえり	腓返り（腓肠肌痉挛）
ごゆけつ	五俞穴
こんけつ	昏厥
こんすい	昏睡
こんだく	混濁
こんろん	崑崙

さ

さいきんせいげり	細菌性下痢
させい	嗄聲（声音嘶哑）
さむがり	寒がり（形寒）
さむけ	寒気（发冷）
さんいん	三陰
さんいんこう	三陰交
さんちく	攢竹
さんりょうしん	三稜針

し

しいん	至陰
じかせんえん	耳下腺炎（腮腺炎）

しきもう	色盲
しきゅうだっすい	子宮脱垂
じけつ	耳穴
しこう	支溝
ししん	指針
ししんそう	四神聡
じしんりょうほう	耳針療法
したいだつりょくかん	肢体脱力感
したがかわき	舌が乾き（舌干）
しつう	歯痛
しつがいこつ	膝蓋骨
しつかきんけいれん	膝窩筋痙攣
じっせん	十宣
じつぜん	実喘
しつねつ	湿熱
しつねつげり	湿熱下痢
じつぴ	実秘
しびれ	痺れ（麻木）
しぶつふめい	視物不明
じめい	耳鳴
じもん	耳門
しゃくたく	尺沢
しゃくねつかん	灼熱感
しゃっくり	吃逆（呃逆）
しゅっしん	出針
じゅんけいしゅけつ	循経取穴
じゅんこう	循行
じゅんこうルート	循行途径
じゅうしけい	十四経

しょうかい	照海
しょうかつ	消渇
しょうかふりょう	消化不良
しょうざん	承山
しょうざんか	焼山火
しょうにきょうふう	小児驚風
じょうしつう	上肢痛
しょうしょう	承漿
しょうしょう	少衝
しょうしょう	少商
じょうせい	上星
しょうたく	少沢
しょうべんがつうじない	小便が通じない（小便不利）
しょうみゃく	衝脈
じょうみゃく	静脈
しょうよう	商陽
しょくせききたい	食積気滞
しょくどうきょうさく	食道狭窄
しょくよくげんたい	食慾減退
しらが	白髪
しらぞこい	白底翳（白内障）
しりょくげんたい	視力減退
しわをよせる	皺を寄せる（皺額）
しんかん	針感
しんき	心悸
じんきょ	腎虚
しんさい	沈細（沉细）
しんし	針刺
しんしますい	針刺麻酔

しんしん	進針
しんじんふこう	心腎不交
しんせん	震顫
しんはん	心煩
じんましん	蕁麻疹
しんもん	神門
しんゆ	心俞
じんゆ	腎俞
じんようふそく	腎陽不足

す

ずい	頭維
すいいんないてい	水飲内停
すいしゅ	水腫
すいしんりょうほう	水針療法

せ

せいけい	正経
せいけつ	井穴
せいしんふしん	精神不振
せいしんぶんれつしょう	精神分裂症
せいちゅう	怔忡
せいめい	睛明
せいりつう	生理痛（痛経）
せき	咳き（咳嗽）
せきちゅうきょうちょく	脊柱強直
せきり	赤痢
ぜっきょうちょく	舌強直
せっしん	折針

ぜつたい	舌苔
ぜんしんそうようかん	全身搔痒感
ぜんそく	喘息
ぜんとうどうちくのうしょう	前頭洞蓄膿症（額窦积脓）
ぜんわんないそくつう	前腕内側痛

そ

ぞうえ	臓会
そうすう	壮数
ぞうそう	臓躁
そくきょういん	足竅陰
そくきょうつう	側胸痛
そくさんり	足三里
そこひ	底翳（目翳）
そこまめ	底豆（鶏眼）
そっちゅうしつご	卒中失語（中风不语）
そっちゅうだっしょう	卒中脱症（中风脱证）
そっちゅうへいしょう	卒中閉症（中风闭证）

た

たいいふせい	胎位不正
たいえん	太淵
たいけい	太谿
たいしゃ	大瀉
たいしょう	太衝
たいしん	体針
たいしん	滞針
たいしん	退針
たいじょうほうしん	帯状疱疹

だいたいないそくつう	大腿内側痛
だいつい	大椎
たいひょう	体表
たいよう	太陽
たいみゃく	帯脈
だっこう	脱肛
だっしょう	脱症
だっちょう	脱腸
たむ	多夢
たんかないどう	痰火内動
たんしつないてい	痰湿内停
だんちゅう	膻中

ち

ちかん	遅緩
ちくでき	抽搐
ちそう	地倉
ちつぺん	秩辺
ちょうかい	聴会
ちょうき	調気
ちょうきゅう	聴宮
ちょうきょう	長強
ちょうこつぜんじょうきょく	腸骨前上棘
ちょうしん	長針
ちょうそう	疔瘡
ちょうめい	腸鳴
ちょうろうぞうせつじゅつ	腸瘻造設術
ちょくせつきゅう	直接灸
ちゅうかん	中脘

ちゅうきょく	中極
ちゅうしょ	中渚
ちゅうしょう	中衝
ちゅうぶこうれん	肘部拘攣
ちんち	沈遅（沉迟）

つ

ついかんばん	椎間盤
ついかんばんヘルニア	椎間盤脱出
ついまひ	対麻痺（双瘫、截瘫）
つうてん	痛点
つうかく	痛覚
つうかくかびん	痛覚過敏
つうふう	痛風
つうふうせいかんせつえん	痛風性関節炎
つうり	通里

て

ていけつあつしょう	低血圧症
ていけっとうショック	低血糖ショック（胰岛素休克）
ていけっとうしょう	低血糖症
ていそう	提挿
ていねい	耵聹
てきちゅう	滴虫
てきおうしょう	適応症
てくびむりょく	手首無力（手腕无力）
てんねんとう	天然痘（天花）
てのけついんしんぽうけい	手厥陰心包経

— 361 —

てのしょういんしんけい	手少陰心経
てのしょうようさんしょうけい	手少陽三焦経
てのたいいんはいけい	手太陰肺経
てのたいようしょうちょうけい	手太陽小腸経
てのみずむし	手の水虫（鵝掌风）
てのようめいだいちょうけい	手陽明大腸経
てんかん	癲癇
てんきょう	癲狂
てんし	点刺
てんしん	転針
でんしん	電針
てんそう	天宗
てんすう	天枢
てんとつ	天突

と

どうき	動悸（心动过速）
どうき	導気
とうけつ	透穴
どうしりょう	瞳子髎
とうしん	透針
とうしん	搗針
とうしんりょうほう	頭針療法
とうてんりょう	透天涼
どうしんすん	同身寸
とくき	得気
とくび	犢鼻
とくみゃく	督脈
とけつ	吐血

としん	兎唇
とさつ	塗擦
とつぜんこんとう	突然昏倒
とりめ	鳥目（夜盲）
とんし	頓死（猝死）

な

ないいん	内因
ないかん	内関
ないてい	内庭
ないぶんぴつ	内分泌
なえる	萎える（癱瘓）
なめらか	滑らか（光滑）
なんちょう	難聴　耳聾
なんべん	軟便

に

にきび	面皰（痤瘡）
にっしゃびょう	日射病（中暑）
にゅうせんえん	乳腺炎
にょうしっきん	尿失禁
にょうへい	尿閉　尿潴留
にんしんおそ	妊娠悪阻
にんちゅう	人中

ね

ねあせ	寝汗（盗汗）
ねんちょう	粘稠
ねしょうべん	寝小便（夜尿）

ねつがでる	熱が出る（发热）
ねんざしょう	扭挫傷
ねんしん	捻針
ねんてんほしゃ	捻転補瀉

の

のど	喉・咽（咽喉）
のどちんこ	喉ちんこ（悬壅垂）
のどぶえ	喉笛（声門）
のどぼとけ	喉仏（喉结）
のみこむ	呑み込む（呑下）
のぼせ	逆上せ（头晕）

は

ばいかしん	梅花針
はいそういんきょ	肺躁陰虚
はいにょうこんなん	排尿困難
はいゆ	背俞
はいゆ	肺俞
はいせきつう	背脊痛
はをくいしばる	歯を食いしばる（牙关紧闭）
はきだす	吐き出す（吐泻）
はくたいげ	白帯下
ばっかかん	抜火罐
ばっかんりょうほう	抜罐療法
はつねつ	発熱（发热）
ばっしん	抜針
はなつまり	鼻詰り（鼻塞）
はなみず	鼻みず（鼻涕）

はり	針
はんかつ	煩渇
はんこんきゅう	瘢痕灸
はんしんふずい	半身不遂
はんそう	煩躁

ひ

ひいきょじゃく	脾胃虚弱
ひきつけ	引き付け（抽搐）
ひきょ	脾虚
ひきょけっしょう	脾虚血少
びけつ	鼻血
ひざ	膝
ひざしゅつう	膝腫痛
ひざとしょうたいのとうつう	膝と小腿の疼痛（膝脛痛）
ひざのいたみ	膝の痛み（膝痛）
ひじかんせつ	肘関節
ひしょう	痺症
ひゆ	脾俞
ひゃくえ	百会
ひんにょう	頻尿

ふ

ふうかん	風寒
ふうし	風市
ふうしん	風疹
ふうち	風池
ふうねつ	風熱
ふうふ	風府

ふえ	腑会
ふきん	浮緊
ふくちょうまんかん	腹脹満感（腹胀）
ふくつう	腹痛
ふくと	伏兎
ふくりゅう	復溜
ふさく	浮数
ふにんしょう	不妊症
ふみん	不眠（失眠）
プローバ	（探針）

へ

へいしょう	閉症
へそ	臍
べつらく	別絡
ヘルニア	疝
べんぴ	便秘

ほ

ほほぼね	頬骨（顴骨）
ぼうまんかん	膨満感（胀満感）
ほうりゅう	豊隆
ほうろう	崩漏
ぼけつ	募穴
ほしゃ	補瀉
ほろし	痱子（蕁麻疹）

ま

まつげ	睫毛

まぶた	眼瞼
まゆげ	眉毛
まゆをひそめる	眉を顰める（蹙眉）
まんきょうふう	慢驚風
マラリヤ	疟疾

み

みっかはしか	風疹
みつくち	三つ口（兔唇）
みみ	耳
みみくそ	耳垢
みみたぶ	耳朵（耳廓）
みみだれ	耳垂れ（耳液溢）
みみなり	耳鳴
みゃくえ	脈会

む

むかん	無汗
むくみ	浮腫（全身水肿）
むしば	齲歯
むせい	夢精
むねやけ	胸焼け（胃灼热感）
むはんこんきゅう	無瘢痕灸

め

めがしら	目頭（内眦）
めいもん	命門
めがあかくはれていたい	目が赤く張れて痛い（目赤肿痛）

めくら	盲
めじり	目尻（外眼角）
めだま	目玉（眼球）
めまい	目眩（眩暈）

も

もうちょうえん	盲腸炎
ものもらい	物貰い（麦粒肿）

や

やくかん	薬罐
やくぶつがいかん	薬物艾巻
やけど	焼傷
やもうしょう	夜盲症

ゆ

ゆうせん	湧泉
ゆびのしびれ	指の痺れ（指端麻木）
ゆめ	夢

よ

よあけまえ	夜明け前（天亮前）
ようつう	腰痛
ようしがだるくてむりょく	腰膝がだるくて無力（腰膝酸软）
ようせんぶつう	腰仙部痛（腰骶痛）
ようはく	陽白
ようめい	陽明
ようりょうせん	陽陵泉

よだれ	涎
よなき	夜泣き（夜啼）

り

りきゅうこうじゅう	裏急後重
リウマチ	風湿
リウマチようかんせつえん	リウマチ様関節炎（类风湿性关节炎）
りゅうしん	留針
りゅうせん	流涎
りゅうへい	癃閉
りゅうるい	流涙
りゅうこうシーズン	流行シーズン（流行季节）
りょう	鬱
りょうきゅう	梁丘
りょうもん	梁門
りんしょう	淋症
りんれき	淋瀝

る

るいれき	瘰癧
るいのうえん	涙嚢炎
るいそう	消痩

れ

れいだ	歷兌
れっけつ	列缺
れんせん	廉泉

ろ

ろうきゅう	労宮
ろうか	老化
ろうねんせいなんちょう	老年性難聴
ろうねんせいちほ	老年性痴呆
ろうねんせいそうようしょう	老年性搔痒症
ろくかんしんけいつう	肋間神経痛
ろくまくえん	肋膜炎（胸膜炎）

わ

わかがえり	若返り（返老还童）
わきが	腋臭
わんかんせつ	腕関節
わんしん	彎針

※（　）内为汉语，无（　）为中日通用汉语。
　（　）内は漢語、（　）のないのは日漢通用なものである。

【附】中文簡化字繁體字對照

二劃
儿〔兒〕
几〔幾〕

三劃
广〔廣〕
干〔乾〕
于〔於〕
亏〔虧〕
卫〔衛〕
习〔習〕
叉〔扠〕
门〔門〕
么〔麼〕
个〔個〕

四劃
为〔爲〕
认〔認〕
开〔開〕
丰〔豐〕
专〔專〕
无〔無〕
区〔區〕

厅〔廳〕
历〔歷〕
扎〔紮〕
书〔書〕
见〔見〕
冈〔岡〕
长〔長〕
从〔從〕
仓〔倉〕
仑〔崙〕
仅〔僅〕
气〔氣〕
风〔風〕
办〔辦〕
双〔雙〕

五劃
头〔頭〕
汇〔滙〕
记〔記〕
术〔術〕
龙〔龍〕
布〔佈〕
厉〔厲〕
对〔對〕

发〔發〕
写〔寫〕
它〔牠〕
宁〔寧〕
节〔節〕
业〔業〕
叶〔葉〕
叹〔嘆〕
归〔歸〕
电〔電〕
册〔冊〕
仪〔儀〕
务〔務〕
饥〔饑〕
处〔處〕

六劃
庆〔慶〕
产〔產〕
齐〔齊〕
关〔關〕
并〔並〕
兴〔興〕
当〔當〕
刘〔劉〕

冲〔衝〕
动〔動〕
壮〔壯〕
论〔論〕
讲〔講〕
设〔設〕
夹〔夾〕
过〔過〕
达〔達〕
压〔壓〕
厌〔厭〕
巩〔鞏〕
扬〔揚〕
寻〔尋〕
导〔導〕
异〔異〕
尽〔盡〕
阴〔陰〕
阳〔陽〕
阵〔陣〕
团〔團〕
贞〔貞〕
师〔師〕
则〔則〕
众〔衆〕

— 371 —

后〔後〕 来〔來〕 闷〔悶〕 拢〔攏〕
欢〔歡〕 两〔兩〕 苏〔蘇〕 现〔現〕
囱〔囪〕 志〔誌〕 余〔餘〕 环〔環〕
负〔負〕 励〔勵〕 肠〔腸〕 郁〔鬱〕
杂〔雜〕 严〔嚴〕 采〔採〕 轮〔輪〕
创〔創〕 麦〔麥〕 乱〔亂〕 软〔軟〕
优〔優〕 折〔摺〕 条〔條〕 转〔轉〕
伤〔傷〕 扰〔擾〕 系〔係〕 肾〔腎〕
华〔華〕 张〔張〕 针〔針〕 齿〔齒〕
纤〔纖〕 进〔進〕 体〔體〕 国〔國〕
妇〔婦〕 还〔還〕 饮〔飲〕 实〔實〕
会〔會〕 迟〔遲〕 审〔審〕
连〔連〕 **八劃** 茎〔莖〕
七劃 远〔遠〕 变〔變〕 范〔範〕
弃〔棄〕 运〔運〕 疟〔瘧〕 畅〔暢〕
应〔應〕 鸡〔鷄〕 疡〔瘍〕 艰〔艱〕
疗〔療〕 陈〔陳〕 单〔單〕 径〔徑〕
这〔這〕 际〔際〕 学〔學〕 征〔徵〕
灿〔燦〕 极〔極〕 泪〔淚〕 饱〔飽〕
冻〔凍〕 怀〔懷〕 泻〔瀉〕 肤〔膚〕
沟〔溝〕 围〔圍〕 泽〔澤〕 胁〔脇〕
沥〔瀝〕 员〔員〕 话〔話〕 练〔練〕
识〔識〕 县〔縣〕 昆〔崑〕 织〔織〕
证〔證〕 时〔時〕 态〔態〕 线〔綫〕
补〔補〕 里〔裏〕 枣〔棗〕 经〔經〕
状〔狀〕 呕〔嘔〕 构〔構〕 备〔備〕
声〔聲〕 听〔聽〕 枢〔樞〕 参〔參〕
块〔塊〕 忡〔憃〕 担〔擔〕 质〔質〕
医〔醫〕 坚〔堅〕 拥〔擁〕

九劃

总〔總〕
姜〔薑〕
类〔類〕
烂〔爛〕
弯〔彎〕
迹〔跡〕
疮〔瘡〕
疠〔癘〕
浊〔濁〕
济〔濟〕
误〔誤〕
说〔説〕
诱〔誘〕
语〔語〕
举〔舉〕
觉〔覺〕
养〔養〕
挟〔挾〕
标〔標〕
轻〔輕〕
临〔臨〕
显〔顯〕
点〔點〕
虽〔雖〕
哑〔啞〕
药〔藥〕
贴〔貼〕

顺〔順〕
骂〔罵〕
带〔帶〕
胆〔膽〕
脉〔脈〕
胫〔脛〕
须〔須〕
独〔獨〕
选〔選〕
适〔適〕
种〔種〕
复〔復〕
绕〔繞〕
蚀〔蝕〕
钢〔鋼〕

十劃

离〔離〕
挛〔攣〕
瘌〔癩〕
涩〔澀〕
准〔準〕
资〔資〕
症〔癥〕
〔證〕
痉〔痙〕
调〔調〕
请〔請〕
烦〔煩〕

础〔礎〕
顾〔顧〕
晕〔暈〕
盐〔鹽〕
损〔損〕
样〔樣〕
恶〔惡〕
耻〔恥〕
热〔熱〕
较〔較〕
剧〔劇〕
验〔驗〕
难〔難〕
窍〔竅〕
紧〔緊〕
脐〔臍〕
脓〔膿〕
脑〔腦〕
脏〔臟〕
爱〔愛〕
称〔稱〕
积〔積〕
笔〔筆〕
蚍〔蚍〕
〔魁〕
皱〔皺〕

十一劃

盖〔蓋〕

痒〔癢〕
聋〔聾〕
据〔據〕
梦〔夢〕
颈〔頸〕
惧〔懼〕
惊〔驚〕
盘〔盤〕
矫〔矯〕
躯〔軀〕
秽〔穢〕
银〔銀〕
续〔續〕

十二劃

痈〔癰〕
湿〔濕〕
联〔聯〕
确〔確〕
颊〔頰〕
属〔屬〕
遗〔遺〕
睑〔瞼〕
践〔踐〕
锈〔銹〕
锁〔鎖〕
犊〔犢〕

十三劃

痹〔痺〕
数〔數〕
誉〔譽〕
嗳〔噯〕

锥〔錐〕
缠〔纏〕

十五劃

聪〔聰〕

嘱〔囑〕
镊〔鑷〕

十六劃

颠〔顚〕

十九劃

髌〔髕〕

实用针灸手册

安酉川　陈方良　张玉娟　编著

吉林科学技术出版社出版
中国长春市斯大林大街102号
长春新华印刷厂印刷
中国长春市吉林大路23号
中国国际图书贸易总公司发行
（中国国际书店）
北京399信箱

1989年（大32开）第一版（中英日对照）
ISBN　7-5384-0351-5/R·58
00620
14-CEJ-2420S